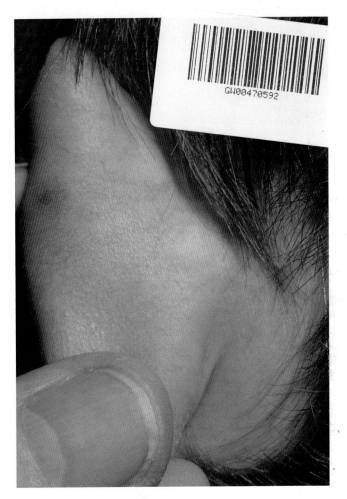

Figure 2.1 Injury to the posterior helix of the ear from a 'pinching' mechanism.

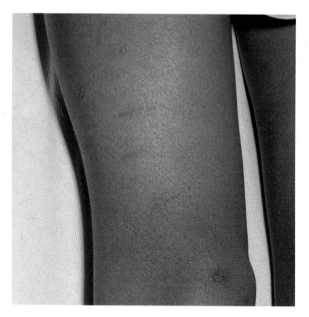

Figure 2.2 Linear marks (scars) to the right thigh.

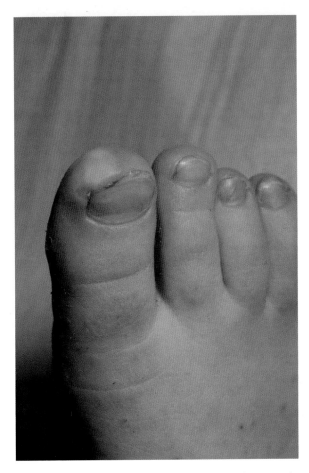

Figure 5.1 Poor foot hygiene with roughly cut nails and blistered great toe from badly fitting shoes.

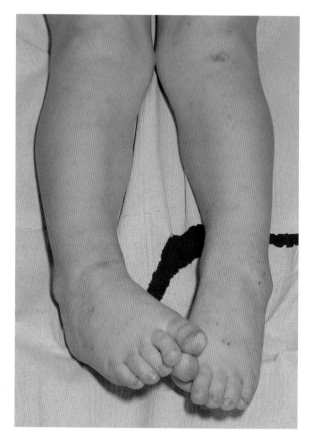

Figure 5.2 Unkempt with multiple scabbed lesions from scabies.

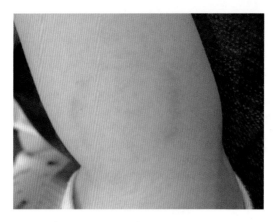

Figure 6.1 Bite to Lisa's forearm as seen at the GP surgery.

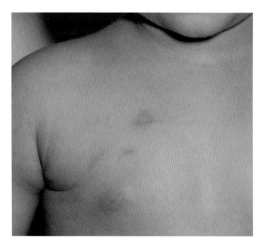

Figure 6.2 Bruises to Luke's chest as seen in the Emergency Department.

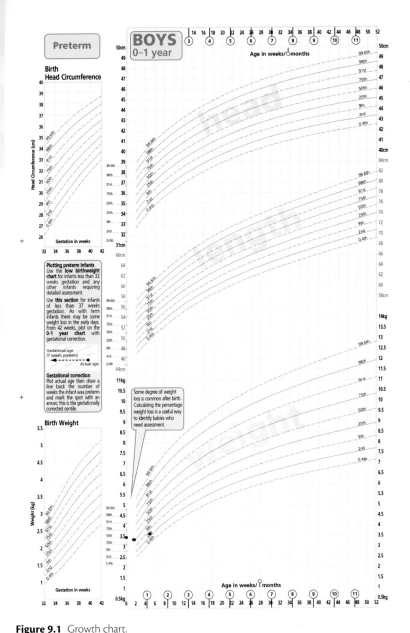

Figure 9.1 Growth chart.

Reproduced with permission from Royal College of Paediatric and Child Health, *Early years - UK-WHO growth charts and resources, Preterm Boys 0-1 year*, UK-WHO Chart 2009, Copyright © DH Copyright 2009, available from http://www.rcpch.ac.uk/system/files/protected/page/A4%20Boys%200-4YRS%20(4th%20Jan%202013).pdf

The grooming line

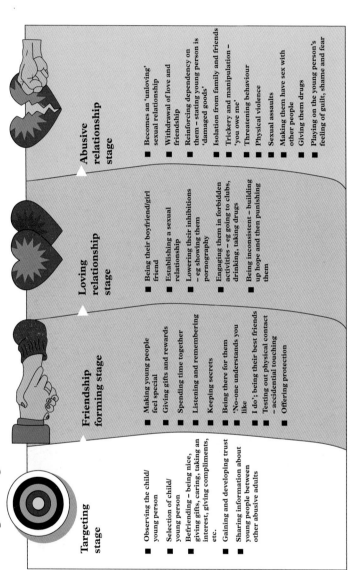

Targeting stage

- Observing the child/young person
- Selection of child/young person
- Befriending – being nice, giving gifts, caring, taking an interest, giving compliments, etc.
- Gaining and developing trust
- Sharing information about young people between other abusive adults

Friendship forming stage

- Making young people feel special
- Giving gifts and rewards
- Spending time together
- Listening and remembering
- Keeping secrets
- Being there for them
- 'No-one understands you like I do'; being their best friends
- Testing out physical contact – accidental touching
- Offering protection

Loving relationship stage

- Being their boyfriend/girl friend
- Establishing a sexual relationship
- Lowering their inhibitions – eg showing them pornography
- Engaging them in forbidden activities – eg going to clubs, drinking, taking drugs
- Being inconsistent – building up hope and then punishing them

Abusive relationship stage

- Becomes an 'unloving' sexual relationship
- Withdrawal of love and friendship
- Reinforcing dependency on them – stating young person is 'damaged goods'
- Isolation from family and friends
- Trickery and manipulation – 'you owe me'
- Threatening behaviour
- Physical violence
- Sexual assaults
- Making them have sex with other people
- Giving them drugs
- Playing on the young person's feeling of guilt, shame and fear

Figure 11.1 The Grooming Line.

The Child
Protection
Practice
Manual

The Child Protection Practice Manual

Training practitioners how to safeguard children

EDITED BY

GAYLE HANN AND CAROLINE FERTLEMAN

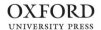

OXFORD
UNIVERSITY PRESS

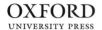

OXFORD
UNIVERSITY PRESS

Great Clarendon Street, Oxford, OX2 6DP,
United Kingdom

Oxford University Press is a department of the University of Oxford.
It furthers the University's objective of excellence in research, scholarship,
and education by publishing worldwide. Oxford is a registered trade mark of
Oxford University Press in the UK and in certain other countries

First Edition published in 2016

Impression: 1

Published in the United States of America by Oxford University Press
198 Madison Avenue, New York, NY 10016, United States of America

British Library Cataloguing in Publication Data
Data available

Library of Congress Control Number: 2015941544

ISBN 978–0–19–870770–7

Printed in Great Britain by
Bell & Bain Ltd., Glasgow

Dedication

In memory of our friend and colleague Michelle Zalkin whose great passion for child protection has inspired many.

This book is dedicated to all the children who have shared their stories with us and changed our lives.

Preface

Child protection is an inherently difficult field as we are taught to believe and listen to the parent. In child protection, this principle has to be set aside, with the child's voice being heard above that of the parent. We must 'think the unthinkable': the parent may be responsible for harming their child.

Around 85 children die every year in the UK due to abuse or neglect. A number of these deaths have been deemed preventable as the families involved were known to either health professionals or social services. High-profile cases have both shocked and distressed the public and highlighted the failings of the very organizations set up to safeguard children.

There is no shortage of overarching principles for what should be done to protect children, but what is missing is a single book that comprehensively covers the child protection process in a practical way. Our book is a training resource for those professionals working in this field, guiding them through the next steps with the use of cases drawn from the authors' experience. We aim for our book to be widely read and indispensible for newcomers and yet still vital for those experienced in the field. We will take readers through the safeguarding process, from how to identify children at risk to appearing as a witness in court, and aim to demystify each step in between. We will also include previously poorly covered territory such as the role of the internet in abuse, child sexual exploitation, trafficking, and gang violence.

This book is predominantly aimed at paediatricians but will prove an equally valuable resource for any professional who comes into contact with children, such as general practitioners, nurses, health visitors, midwives, teachers, lawyers, community workers, and religious leaders. We offer practical advice on documenting accurately and on writing police and court reports, as well as an approach to talking to parents and answering frequently asked questions. Finally, we include new gender-specific anatomically positioned body maps of infants, toddlers, young children, and teenagers to help improve medical record keeping. As authors of this practical guide, we hope to break the complicated safeguarding process into palatable and informative sections that can be read in a few sittings or just returned to for advice.

Please note that, unless otherwise stated, all cases described in this book are fictional, and therefore do not breach any individual's or family's confidentiality, but are constructed to be realistic based on the collective experiences of the authors. Unfortunately, many children are the victims of abuse and therefore the fictional cases used may bear some resemblance to real cases of abuse. Any similarities in names or details are purely coincidental. Any photographs or X-rays that accompany a case have been published with the child's and family's consent.

Acknowledgements

In addition to the authors of the contributing chapters, the editors would like to thank the following people:

Ian Abernethy

Antony Aston

Janet Black-Heaven

Justin Daniels

Louise Day

Sarah Eisen

Hannah Jacob

Christina Keating

Laura Hayman

Linda Helliar

Martin Mensik

Anita Morgan

Cat Parker

Alexandra Perkins

Cisel Ozbay

Claire Rohan

Sarah Stoll

We would also like to thank Conrad von Stempel for his hard work and artistic skills in producing the new body maps.

Thanks are also due to the child protection team at North Middlesex University Hospital (Justin Daniels, Julie Dennehy, Glenda Griffiths, Chantel Palmer, Changu Tsiga, and Debbie Twist), and to Caroline Smith, Nicola Wilson, Camilla Crask and Charlotte Green at Oxford University Press.

Contents

List of contributors

Bryony Alderman
Final Year Medical Student,
University College London Medical
School

Karen Aucott
Paediatric Registrar, Nottingham
University Hospitals NHS Trust

Eleanor Beagley
Final Year Medical Student,
University College London Medical
School

Nirit Braha
Paediatric Registrar, Whittington
Hospital, London

Ellie Day
Paediatric Registrar, St Peter's
Hospital, Chertsey

Katherine Fawbert
Paediatric Registrar and Fellow in
Medical Education, London School
of Paediatrics

Caroline Fertleman
Consultant Paediatrician,
Whittington Hospital, London
Site Subdean for University College
London Medical School at the
Whittington Campus
Honorary Senior Lecturer at the
University College London Institute
of Child Health
Honorary Consultant Paediatrician
at Great Ormond Street Hospital

Christopher Hands
Paediatric Registrar, Imperial
College Healthcare Trust
Charity worker, Klevis Kola
Foundation and Moroccan
Children's Trust

Gayle Hann
Consultant Paediatrician, Named
Doctor, and Lead for Paediatric
Emergency Medicine, North
Middlesex University Hospital
Honorary Senior Lecturer at the
University College London Institute
of Child Health

Laura Haynes
Final Year Medical Student,
University College London Medical
School

Charlotte Holland
Paediatric Registrar, Hackney
Community Health

Maryam Hyrapetian
Paediatric Registrar, Whittington
Hospital, London

Hannah Jacob
Paediatric Registrar, Homerton
Hospital NHS Foundation Trust,
London

David James
Paediatric Registrar and Fellow in
Medical Education, London School
of Paediatrics

Sophie Khadr
Clinical Lecturer, Institute of Child
Health, University College London

Jacqueline Le Geyt
Paediatric Registrar, North
Middlesex University Hospital NHS
Trust, London

Chloe Macaulay
Consultant Paediatrician, Evelina
Children's Hospital, Guys and
St Thomas's NHS Trust

Benita Morrissey
Paediatric Registrar, Whittington
Hospital and Fellow in Medical
Education, University College
London

Eleanor Perera
Paediatric Registrar,
Barnet and Chase Farm
Hospitals NHS Trust,
Hertfordshire

Philippa Prentice
Department of Paediatrics,
University of Cambridge

Kerry Robinson
Consultant Paediatrician,
Whittington Hospital,
London

Arabella Simpkin
Paediatric Registar, Barnet and
Chase Farm Hospitals
NHS Trust,
Hertfordshire

Katherine Taylor
Paediatric Registrar,
Barts and the London
NHS Trust

Conrad von Stempel
Radiology Registrar, University
College Hospital, London

List of body maps

1

The history of child protection and child abuse in the UK. How did we get here?

Philippa Prentice

Chapter summary

Today, protecting children is a priority shared by cultures and societies across the globe. However, the history of child protection, with its legislation, guidelines, and societal norms, is relatively recent. Society, which has not previously considered that children are abused, now deems that its role is to protect them. This chapter will summarize the history of child protection, focusing on the UK. It will briefly describe a time before organized child protection, the origin of child protection societies, and more recent child protection cases, inquiries, and legislation.

Child abuse and protection today

The UN Convention on the Rights of the Child states that every child has the right to a childhood, the right to be educated, the right to be healthy, the right to be treated fairly, and the right to be heard. Of course, child abuse is not confined to the past. The most recent National Society for Prevention of Cruelty to Children (NSPCC) report (April 2013, pp.20, 24) states that, in the UK between 2011 and 2012, there were over 20,000 sexual offences against children and nearly 8,000 cruelty and neglect offences (Harker et al., 2013). Nearly one in five of the young people questioned reported experiencing high levels of abuse or neglect. The report also highlights changing patterns of child abuse over time, with alterations in recognition, reporting, and public awareness. The child homicide rate is declining, as are recorded cases of physical and sexual abuse. However, the number of referrals to children's social services is increasing, with neglect most frequently reported. New patterns of abuse are being seen with one in 13 children of secondary school age reporting persistent cyber bullying and abuse through social networking sites.

History

The history of child protection can be divided into three separate eras (Myers, 2008), summarized for the UK in this section. The history of wider global child protection legislation is well described in a recent review (Cutland, 2012). Box 1.1 summarizes the history of child abuse recognition and different categories of abuse.

Box 1.1 The history of child abuse recognition

Physical abuse

This was first described in the literature as the 'battered child syndrome' and presented as a significant cause of morbidity and mortality in young children (Kempe et al., 1962). This resulted in physical abuse being recognized by medical professionals and then by society. This description followed several other publications suggesting patterns of abuse, for example 'Multiple fractures in the long bones of infants suffering from chronic subdural hematoma' (Caffey, 1946), which introduced the concept of non-accidental injury, 'parent–infant stress syndrome', and the 'shaken baby syndrome'.

Neglect

Kempe was also a pioneer of work in the recognition and description of child neglect.

Sexual abuse

The first description of child sexual abuse was probably given in *Medical–Legal Studies of Sexual Assault (Etude Médico-Légale sur les Attentats aux Moeurs)* by Auguste Ambroise Tardieu in 1857. It was also discussed in the 1890s by Sigmund Freud, who believed that neuroses and mental health conditions were a result of sexual abuse in childhood. However, Freud and others later rejected this theory, and it was not until the 1970s and 1980s that, with the rise of feminism and reports of violence against women, sexual abuse became recognized once more. Before this time there had been occasional criminal proceedings, but cases were normally kept secret, with little public awareness.

Emotional abuse only became increasingly recognized in the 1980s and 1990s.

Munchausen's syndrome by proxy/fabricated and induced illness, described by Meadow in 1977, has only recently been included in child protection manuals.

Early history: no organized child protection, before the mid to late nineteenth century

Throughout history, child labour and neglect have been accepted in the context of poverty and societal structure. It was not seen as society's role to interfere within families, and early examples of helping children in need were limited to the goodwill of a few and mainly to the church. The first laws to focus on rights for children were mainly the result of campaigns by philanthropists to limit working hours for children in factories, chimneys and mines in the 1800s. At this time, child labour was common, schooling was inadequate, and child mortality was high, with child abuse often unrecognized. Many authors of the time portrayed the child's place in society, such as Dickens, who had himself been sent to a workhouse at a young age and was an advocate for better working conditions.

From the late nineteenth century to the mid twentieth century: the origin of child protection societies, and increased public awareness

Case 1.1 Ten-year-old Mary Ellen and the first child protection society

Mary Ellen Wilson was born in 1864 in New York City. After her father died, and her mother's finances meant that she could not afford to pay for some-one to look after Mary Ellen, she was sent to the Department of Charities for adoption. Mary Ellen experienced continued physical abuse and neglect by her carers. She was regularly beaten, forced to do labour, and neglected both phys-ically and emotionally. Her neighbours were aware of Mary Ellen's suffering and enlisted the help of a local Methodist mission worker, Etta Wheeler, and subsequently Henry Bergh.

Changes to legislation

Mary Ellen's case was taken to the New York State Supreme Court in 1874 by Henry Bergh. At the time there was little formal child protection legislation and authorities had been reluctant to intervene. However, Bergh had previ-ously founded the Society for the Prevention of Cruelty to Animals and was now compelled to campaign for Mary Ellen. He was successful, and went on to establish the first child protection society—the New York Society for the Prevention of Cruelty to Children—in 1875.

After visiting the USA, Thomas Agnew set up the first UK society. The local Society for the Prevention of Cruelty to Children began in Liverpool in 1883 and combined with its London counterpart to form the NSPCC in 1889. The NSPCC was instrumental in changing legislation and society's views and expectations. Lobbying efforts resulted in the Children's Charter

(1889), the first Act of Parliament in the UK to protect children. This allowed the law to intervene between parents and their children, and to arrest anyone mistreating a child. It was the start of a succession of acts protecting children, including the Prevention of Cruelty to Children Act and the Children and Young Persons Act.

Recent history: the current era of government child protection services

More recently, the majority of changes in the child protection field have been catalysed by individual cases. In the last 70 years, there have been more than 70 child protection government inquiries and multiple changes to legislation.

Case 1.2 Twelve-year-old Dennis O'Neill and care for looked after children

Dennis was a 12-year-old Welsh boy who had been moved to out-of-area foster care in Shropshire with his younger brother in the middle of 1944. He died in January 1945 after being beaten on his chest and back with a stick. He was found to be severely undernourished, with infected ulcers on his legs and markings of being repetitively beaten. No inquiry had been made into the suitability of the foster care placement of Dennis and his brother, and they had no regular visits or medical reviews.

Changes to legislation

Dennis's death whilst in foster care led to one of the first child protection inquiries, the Monckton Report (1945), which resulted in new legislation for looked after children, such as formation of a committee to find and supervise foster care placements and the need for regular medical examinations and supervision. It subsequently led to the Children Act 1948. A more integrated service for looked after children was established, and specific local authority departments with children's officers were designated for caring for these children.

In 1970, under the Local Authority Social Services Act, local authority social work services and all other social care provisions were amalgamated into social services departments. In 1973 seven-year-old Maria Colwell died as a result of physical abuse by her stepfather. Following her death and a subsequent inquiry, area child protection committees were established. This meant that representatives from all main agencies worked together to safeguard children in a geographical area, improving multidisciplinary responsibility. The 'at-risk register' was also established at this time.

Many other high-profile cases followed in the 1980s and 1990s, all children abused or neglected by adults with parental responsibility, from Heidi Koseda (1984), a three-year-old starved to death, to Chelsea Brown (1999), a two-year-old battered to death. All of these children had been under the care of, referred to, or known to social care. In the midst of these cases, two important child protection developments took place:

Children Act 1989 This is still the basis of the child protection system in England and Wales. It is summarized by its title: 'An Act to reform the law relating to children; to provide for local authority services for children in need and others; to amend the law with respect to children's homes, community homes, voluntary homes and voluntary organizations; to make provision with respect to fostering, child minding and day care for young children and adoption; and for connected purposes'.

Cleveland Inquiry 1988 This investigated a dramatic increase in reported child abuse cases in Cleveland, leading to a crisis in social care placements and a breakdown in the working relationship between social workers, police, and medical professionals, as well as public criticism and lack of concern for the rights of parents. Over a hundred children had been diagnosed as having been sexually abused, many due to the finding of anal dilatation alone, and many were removed from their homes. The inquiry once again concluded that multi-agency communication must improve, and that agencies need to work together, with no one professional diagnosing sexual abuse alone.

Case 1.3 Victoria Climbié and the Laming Report

Victoria Adjo Climbié was born on 2 November 1991 near Abidjan in the Ivory Coast. She came to London in April 1999 with her great-aunt Marie-Therese Kouao, travelling with a passport in the name and photo of another child 'Anna' and wearing a wig over a shaven head. Towards the end of her life, Victoria was tied up inside a black plastic sack in the bath and forced to eat cold food from a piece of plastic. She died 11 months later, and at post-mortem was found to have 128 separate injuries. Victoria and Kouao had been known to at least three housing authorities, four social care departments, including receiving home visits, two child protection teams from the Metropolitan Police service, a specialist centre managed by the NSPCC, and GP surgeries. Victoria had also been admitted to two hospitals with suspected abuse in July 1999: she was taken to the Central Middlesex Hospital by the daughter of her unregistered child minder, with injuries to her fingers and a swollen face, and to the North Middlesex Hospital by Kouao, with a serious scald to the face and other marks on her body.

Changes to legislation

The Laming Report (2003) concluded that over a period of 10 months at least 12 opportunities to save Victoria were missed by social services, police, and NHS professionals. Laming stated that '. . . the suffering and death of Victoria was a gross failure of the system and was inexcusable'. The report described a consistent absence of good practice, organizational failures, unclear responsibility at multiple levels, unallocated child in need cases, and 'under-resourced, understaffed, under-managed, dysfunctional' social care departments. Recommendations included essential multi-agency working, the importance of case recording, appropriate training and responsibility, communication, and supervision by directors and managers of social care. Suggestions were made for better communication between and within social care teams, including handovers, referrals confirmed in writing within 48 hours, and each local authority having a free 24-hour telephone referral number. Before closing a case it was seen as essential to have seen and spoken to the child and the child's carers, and also that the living environment had been visited, views of all involved professionals obtained, and a plan made.

The government green paper *Every Child Matters* (2003) and the Children Act 2004 followed the Laming Report, emphasizing a child-focused approach and multi-agency working, and reflecting many of the recommendations made by Lord Laming. *Every Child Matters* found that the following five outcomes mattered most to children and young people: being healthy, staying safe, enjoying and achieving, making a positive contribution, and economic well-being.

Other consequences included the creation of a government Children and Families Board, the appointments of Margaret Hodge as the first children's minister in 2003 and Professor Al Aynsley-Green as England's first children's commissioner in 2005. Statutory Local Safeguarding Children Boards replaced Area Child Protection Committees, new initiatives such as Sure Start were brought in to support parents, reforms were made to the youth justice system, and investment in adolescent mental health services was increased, all of which had the potential to improve child protection.

Case 1.4 Peter Connelly and *Working Together*

Peter died in 2007 at 17 months of age as a result of physical injuries including a broken back and broken ribs. As with others, he had been known to many agencies, including housing departments, social care, and several hospitals. He was subject to a child protection plan for physical abuse and neglect, after presenting to hospital with a head injury and bruising consistent with non-accidental injury. Because of the extent of concern for his welfare, Peter was put into the care of a family friend but later returned home to his mother. The day before his death he was seen by a community paediatrician for a developmental assessment, where physical abuse with extensive injuries was most likely undetected. Notably, like Victoria Climbié, Peter Connelly had lived in the London Borough of Haringey and was known to social care there. Peter's mother, her boyfriend, and his brother were all convicted of causing or allowing Peter's death.

Changes to legislation

Inquiries followed, including a further report from Lord Laming, *The Protection of Children in England: A Progress Report* (2009). Many of his previous recommendations were re-emphasized, including multi-agency working, the importance of leadership, accountability, and responsibility, and collaboration up to government level, including the establishment of the National Safeguarding Delivery Unit (2009).

Since the death of Peter Connelly, new statutory guidance has been published in *Working Together to Safeguard Children* (2010, updated in 2013). This outlines how organizations and individuals should work together to safeguard and promote the welfare of children and young people in accordance with the Children Acts 1989 and 2004. Key messages from this document include a child-centred and coordinated approach to safeguarding, with early help and information sharing. It emphasizes that safeguarding is *everyone's responsibility* at the individual and organizational level, including the NHS, police, schools, and youth offending teams. There are clear guidelines for referrals, assessment, child protection plans, and conferences, and information about what to do when things go wrong.

Another important recent review of child protection practice is Professor Eileen Munro's independent review of child protection in England, *A Child-centred System*, published in 2011 and updated in 2012. Munro's report made 15 recommendations focusing on reducing the amount of 'box-ticking' and blindly following procedures and rules, whilst increasing focus on the needs and experiences of individual children.

Other aspects of child protection history

Alongside new legislation and recommendations, there have recently been important changes to child protection training and advances in research. In 2003 the Royal College of Paediatrics and Child Health began a project to develop child protection training, after an NSPCC survey of training needs in child protection for paediatrics showed that this was a priority. Further information on child protection training can be found in Chapter 20 and on the Royal College of Paediatrics and Child Health website (http://www.rcpch.ac.uk/).

Child protection research is still relatively new but has helped to shape the history of this field. Large systematic reviews have been instrumental in forming and changing guidelines. The Cardiff Core Info system (http://www.core-info.cardiff.ac.uk) has provided an invaluable source of information for all paediatricians working in the child protection field.

Conclusion

The history of child protection shows the significant changes in legislation, responsibility, and societal involvement in the care of children in need during the last century. Serious child protection cases, their consequences, and inspirational leaders have driven the development of child protection services, new legislation, and guidelines. Multiple inquiries and reports highlight the importance of efficient communication, coordination with multi-agency working, appropriate documentation, and taking responsibility at all levels. Perhaps most importantly, recent recommendations are for a child-centred approach, listening to our children and acting on their behalf. The future will be shaped by new cases, reports, and legislation, but also by the changing nature of society, communication, and the media.

References

Caffey, J. (1946). Multiple fractures in the long bones of infants suffering from chronic subdural hematoma. *Radiology*, **194**, 163–73.

Cutland, M. (2012). Child abuse and its legislation: the global picture. *Archives of Disease in Childhood*, **97**(8), 679–84.

Harker, L., Jütte, S., Murphy, T., Bentley, H., Miller, P., Fitch, K. (2013). *How Safe Are Our Children?* NSPCC report. Available at: www.nspcc.org.uk/Inform/research/findings/howsafe/how-safe-2013-report_wdf95435.pdf.

Kempe, C.H., Silverman, F.N., Steele, B.F., Droegemuller, W., Silver, H.K. (1962) The battered child syndrome. *Journal of the American Medical Association*, **181**, 17–24.

Laming Report (2003). *The Victoria Climbié Inquiry*. Available at: http://www.official-documents.gov.uk/document/cm57/5730/5730.pdf (accessed 10 September 2014).

Meadow, R. (1977). Munchausen syndrome by proxy. The hinterland of child abuse. *Lancet*, **2**(8033), 343–5.

Myers, J.E.B. (2008). A short history of child protection in America. *Family Law Quarterly*, **42**(3), 449–63.

Tardieu, A.A. (1857). Etude Médico-légale sur les Attentats aux Moeurs. (Medical–Legal Studies of Sexual Assault). Paris: Librairie JB Baillière et Fils.

2

Child protection and the law

Gayle Hann

Chapter summary

The UK has a complex collection of acts and guidance under constant revision covering child protection rather than a single law. As a result, health professionals and the general public may get confused as to what constitutes child abuse, particularly physical abuse. The variation in legislation for England, Wales, Scotland, and Northern Ireland will be discussed as well as gaps in the law, such as the minimum age for a babysitter and at what age a child can be left alone. The cases presented have been chosen to cover the current laws relating to children as well as to highlight common legal and ethical dilemmas that are often faced in child protection work.

Case 2.1 The child protection framework

You are the paediatric registrar on call seeing Jasmine, six years old, who presents with recurrent abdominal pain. The emergency doctor is concerned that Jasmine did not make any eye contact or speak during the consultation. You examine Jasmine and can find no obvious cause for her abdominal pain, but notice a 1 cm circular bruise with a central area of skin loss on the rim of her left ear (see Figure 2.1).

You ask Jasmine what happened to her ear, but she doesn't speak and just stares at her mother, Rosemary. Her mother reports that she is very noisy at home. You have found it difficult to take a social history as Jasmine's 18-month-old brother, Thomas, is jumping around and shouting. Jasmine's mother calls her nine-year-old daughter, Isabel, from the waiting room to take him out to play. You notice that Isabel has a bruise beneath her right eye (see Chapter 17, 'How will you record Isabel's injuries?'). When you ask Rosemary what happened she reports that her toddler, Thomas, hit Isabel with a cup.

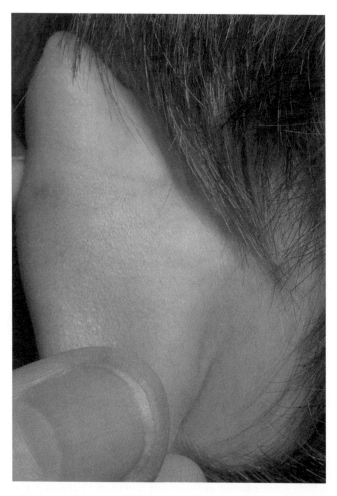

Figure 2.1 Injury to the posterior helix of the ear from a 'pinching' mechanism (see also colour plate section).

You explain to Rosemary that you wish to carry out further investigations. You start by collecting a urine sample and routine blood tests and plotting Jasmine's growth. You check to see if the children are subject to a child protection plan (formerly known as being on the child protection register) and phone social care to see if the family is known. The children are not on a plan but have had a previous assessment six months ago due to domestic violence.

Case 2.1 Exercise

◆ What are your concerns?

◆ Are there any risk factors for child protection?

◆ With regard to the law, what legislation exists to protect these children?

◆ What are the responsibilities of the agencies involved in this case?

Case 2.1 Discussion

What are your concerns?

Physical abuse is possible. All injuries and any concerns should be examined in context. Lacerations are the most common type of accidental ear injury and occur most frequently in males (Steele and Brennan, 2002). In this case, the bruise to the ear and the other child protection risk factors listed should sound alarm bells. Recurrent abdominal pain can suggest a non-organic cause if all other investigations are normal. As Case 2.1 evolves, the mother later admits to pulling Jasmine out of bed by her ear.

Are there any risk factors for child protection?

Yes, there are several. Potential risk factors will be described further in Chapter 5, but pertinent to this case are:

◆ Elective mutism and poor eye contact can suggest abuse. Jasmine's behaviour also has some elements of frozen watchfulness. Elective mutism, often attributed to defiance or emotional trauma, has many causes (Hayden, 1980). All behaviours should be taken in context and mutism should be seen as a piece of the jigsaw when other risk factors are present. Further evaluation of Jasmine is warranted.

◆ A second child in the family with a facial bruise (Isabel's black eye) should make you look closer by taking a detailed family and social history.

◆ The fact that Thomas was reported to have caused the black eye by hitting his sister Isabel with a cup is concerning, as blaming siblings for injuries is an unfortunate known occurrence in cases of non-accidental injury. An 18-month-old would not usually be able to reach a nine-year-old's face or throw a cup with enough force to cause such an injury. The mechanism should be explored further and any inconsistencies in the story noted.

◆ There has been a previous history of domestic violence within the family—this will be covered further in Chapters 8 and 9.

With regard to the law, what legislation exists to protect these children?

There is much legislation in existence to protect the children involved in this case. The current legal framework for England and Wales is based on the Children Act 1989 which included the principles listed in Box 2.1. Its evolution is described in Chapter 1.

As covered in Chapter 1, the law was revised in the Children Act 2004 as a response to the findings of Lord Laming's inquiry into the death of Victoria Climbié. All agencies must have:

◆ robust procedures for information sharing

◆ managers committed to children's welfare and well-being

◆ a clear line of accountability for work on safeguarding

Box 2.1 Principles of the Children Act 1989

1) The child's welfare must come first ('paramountcy').
2) Significant harm is the threshold which justifies compulsory intervention in family life.
3) Parents have a duty to act responsibly with regard to the welfare of their children and local authorities have a duty to support them to do this.
4) Local authorities are to identify children in need and to safeguard and promote their welfare.
5) Social care are responsible for investigating child protection concerns and should work in partnership with parents whenever possible.
6) Children should have a say in what happens to them within legal proceedings.
7) A checklist of factors should be considered by the court before reaching decisions.
8) Delays should be avoided when reaching court decisions as they are likely to be harmful to the child's welfare.

- clear procedures in place for checking that staff are safe to work with children (Criminal Records Bureau checks which were replaced by the Disclosure and Barring Service in April 2013)

- staff with the appropriate training in child protection.

There is very little difference between the frameworks used in England, Wales, Scotland, and Northern Ireland. The Children Acts 1989 and 2004 cover England and Wales. Should you wish to read further, the laws are the Children (Scotland) Act 1995 and the Children (Northern Ireland) Order 1995, which share the same principles and have their own guidance.

The family in Case 2.1 previously came to the attention of social services for domestic violence. Although it is not stated, it was likely that this was reported by a health professional. The Domestic Violence, Crime and Victims Act 2004 also exists to protect children, and this will be covered further in Chapter 8. As Case 2.1 evolves in chapters 16 and 17, the principles of the Children Acts 1989 and 2004 will come to life.

What are the responsibilities of the individuals and agencies involved in this case?

The triage nurse Under the guidance of the Royal College of Nursing (RCN, 2007), the triage nurse has a responsibility to report any concerns she has to social care. She can do this without the agreement of the doctor, although it is best practice to work as a team and share information.

The doctor It is the responsibility of the doctor, under the guidance of the General Medical Council (GMC, 2012) to escalate any child protection concerns. We recommend that junior doctors discuss all concerns with the paediatric team before discharging a child and that the paediatric consultant on duty is informed of all children referred to social care.

The hospital Until 1974, hospitals employed their own social workers. With recent health and social care reforms as described in chapter 1, the responsibility has shifted to local authorities. As previously stated, it is the duty of the hospital to ensure that their staff are appropriately trained in recognizing and responding to safeguarding concerns, have robust child protection policies, a named doctor and nurse for child protection, and a referral framework that allows open communication and the flow of information with partner agencies.

Social care Under the Children Act 1989, the responsibility to protect children falls to local authorities and family courts, and therefore once a referral is made to social care, it is their duty to investigate and act upon their concerns. This responsibility was highlighted in the failures of Haringey social services in the case of Peter Connelly ('Baby P') and led to the recommendations made in the Munro Review (Munro, 2011).

Case 2.1 Summary

With regard to what the doctor should do in Case 2.1, there is more than one correct answer, but we recommend that a discussion is held with a social worker (duty team if out of hours) followed by a written referral (typically by email or fax), and that a rapid assessment of the family is made by social care. This may involve admitting Jasmine whilst further enquiries are made with the GP, health visitor, and school nurse. The social worker may wish to hold a strategy meeting including the police's Child Abuse Investigation Team and any other professionals involved with the family. This process will be discussed in Chapter 16.

Case 2.2 The law on physical chastisement

Ten-year-old Olu was noted to have linear marks on both thighs when he attended the GP surgery for a tetanus booster (see Figure 2.2). The practice nurse had asked him how they had occurred but he refused to say what had happened. The nurse asked the GP to take a look who also felt that the marks were suspicious, especially with no explanation. His mother, Toyin, tells the

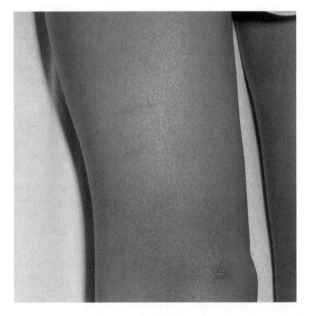

Figure 2.2 Linear marks (scars) to the right thigh (see also colour plate section).

GP that she had caned him for taking money from her purse. She reports that when she was a child in Nigeria, her mother had physically chastised her and that she would be made to pick a branch from a bush to be hit with. She said that it had never done her any harm and many of her friends physically chastise their children. The GP has known the family for many years and has never had any previous concerns. Olu has two siblings, 15-year-old Akin and four-year-old Adeole. Both parents work in the family-owned catering business.

Case 2.2 Exercise

◆ What should the GP do in this case?

◆ Is this child being abused?

◆ What is the law on physical chastisement?

Case 2.2 Discussion

What should the GP do in this case?

There is no single correct answer in this case. The GP has the difficult task of confronting different attitudes towards discipline, some of which may be cultural in origin (see Chapter 12). However, it is illegal in the UK to use an implement to hit a child and therefore a social care referral is warranted. The GP may want to talk to Olu on his own first and find out how frequently and for what reason this discipline is meted out and whether the other children in the family suffer the same fate for misbehaviour. Social care are likely to talk to school teachers or any other agencies involved with the family and arrange Section 47 medicals on all three children (see Chapters 15 and 16 for more details on assessing children for whom there are safeguarding concerns and the safeguarding process).

Is this child being abused?

There is considerable social research in this area. Deater-Deckard and Dodge (1997) argue that punishment has different meanings for some cultural groups. They contend that in cultures where physical punishment is a predominant mode of discipline and is used in a controlled fashion in the context of a nurturing relationship, it is looked on as a sign of good parenting. However, there is much evidence to the contrary. In a meta-analysis Gershoff (2002) found that parental corporal punishment is associated with:

◆ child delinquency

◆ decreased quality of relationship between parent and child

◆ child mental health problems as well as mental health problems as an adult

◆ increased risk of being a victim of physical abuse

◆ increased adult aggression

◆ increased adult criminal and antisocial behaviour

◆ increased risk of abusing their own child or spouse.

In this case, this child has been disciplined in a way that has left marks and considerable pain would have been inflicted along with the physical injury, which would meet the Children Act (1989) definition of ill-treatment.

What is the law on physical chastisement?

The law in England and Wales allows a parent to physically chastise their child as long as it is 'reasonable'. Section 58 of the Children Act 2004 removed the defence of 'reasonable chastisement' for any child punishment that caused such injuries as bruising, swelling, cuts, grazes, or scratches. However, a legal loophole identified by the Sentencing Guidelines Council in 2008 allows parents charged with assault to claim as mitigating circumstances that they intended to punish their child but did not intend to cause bodily harm. The European Court of Human Rights has found UK laws to be in breach of both the European Social Charter and the UN Convention on the Rights of the Child which effectively prohibits all corporal punishment.

Since October 1993, it has been illegal in Scotland to punish children by shaking, hitting on the head, or using a belt, cane, slipper, wooden spoon, or other implement. The law in Northern Ireland is the same as that for England and Wales under Section 58 of the Children Act 2004, except under Article 2 of the Law Reform (Miscellaneous Provisions) (Northern Ireland) Order 2006 which prevents the defence of reasonable chastisement in serious cases of injury to the child such as wounding or grievous bodily harm.

Case 2.2 Summary

Olu's mother has left marks and used an implement which is illegal under the Children Act 2004, but the 'smacking' debate continues in England. Whilst physical punishment of children is banned in 23 countries across the world, it is still a grey area in the UK. This leaves children such as Olu vulnerable to physical abuse under the umbrella of 'reasonable chastisement'. Although the UK legal system is slow to change, we as health professionals must not be slow to act to protect children from harm.

Case 2.3 The law on looking after children whilst intoxicated

You are a junior doctor in the minor injuries unit. George, a lively two-year-old, is brought to the Emergency Department by his mother, Kate, after he tripped and fell, hitting his chin on the pavement. The triage nurse reports that she thought George's mother smelt of alcohol. George's chin has a small laceration and grazes consistent with falling over. His mother appeared to slur her words when you ask her what happened. It is three o'clock in the afternoon and you ask her if she has been drinking. She reports meeting friends for lunch and having a glass of wine.

Case 2.3 Exercise

- What do you do?
- What does the law say about looking after children whilst intoxicated?

Case 2.3 Discussion

What do you do?

George's mother appears to be intoxicated and admits to drinking some alcohol, though not enough to have made her drunk. A full family and social history needs to be taken. A period of observation of George would be reasonable until his mother is sober whilst a discussion is held with the social work team or duty social worker if out of hours. It is important to tell George's mother that you are making a social care referral (see Case 2.4). It would not be helpful in this case to involve the police if you expect to gain a full history and help the family, but you could fall back on this should she refuse to cooperate and try to leave with George. George's needs are paramount in this case and a confrontational approach is rarely helpful.

What does the law say about looking after children whilst intoxicated?

Under Section 1 (2) of the Licensing Act 1902 it is an offence to be drunk whilst in charge of a child under seven years of age in a public place. The same applies for a child under the age of 10 years in Scotland (Section 50 (2) of the Civic Government (Scotland) Act 1982). Neither of these laws makes it an offence to be in charge of a minor in a private place, such as the home. However, under Section 1 of the Children and Young Persons Act 1933 parents who are incapacitated through drink could be charged with neglecting or exposing their child in a manner likely to cause unnecessary suffering or injury to health.

Case 2.3 Summary

It is necessary to stress that being drunk in charge of a child is not in itself child abuse; for that there needs to be exposure to significant harm or specific risk. The key factors in determining the degree of risk will tend to be issues such as the age of the children, proximity to hazards, household circumstances, and frequency and duration of behaviour. However, frequent heavy drinking is harmful as the adult is likely to be neglecting the child's needs and putting them at risk of injury due to a lack of attentiveness during supervision.

Case 2.4 Sharing information where you are concerned that a child or young person is at risk

Mary, the mother of 18-month-old Kevin, is upset because social care have been informed about a burn to his hand. The doctor made a referral to social services as he was concerned that Mary did not adequately supervise her children. She is a single parent who has three children all under the age of five, one of whom, Harley, suffered a recent head injury when he fell out of a window.

Case 2.4 Exercise

♦ Did the GP have a legal duty to inform Mary that he was making the referral?

Case 2.4 Discussion

Did the GP have a legal duty to inform Mary that he was making the referral?

In this case, it would be best for the doctor to seek consent from the mother before sharing information with social services 'unless there is a compelling reason for not doing so' such as:

◆ a delay in sharing relevant information with an appropriate person or authority would increase the risk of harm to the child or young person

◆ asking for consent might increase the risk of harm to the child or young person, or to anyone else (General Medical Council, 2012).

When asking for consent, the doctor should explain what information will shared, who it will be shared with, and how the information will be used.

Case 2.4 Summary

There has been a recent landmark case where a couple brought a case against Haringey social services for conducting a child protection enquiry without informing them that they were under investigation. This has led to social care refusing to conduct enquiries in such instances as described in this case. In the case discussed here the GP has chosen not to inform the parent and therefore should have clearly documented the reasons why they had felt unable to gain consent for the referral.

Case 2.5 Minimum age for babysitting and what age children can be left alone

A mother, Janine, attends the emergency department with her two-year-old son Riley who has a cough and fever. During the course of the consultation, you find out that she is a single parent with four children, the eldest of whom, Kyron, is 14 years old. Kyron has been left looking after the other two children, Cheyanne, aged six, and Tyler, aged four.

Case 2.5 Exercise

◆ Is Janine doing anything wrong by leaving Kyron supervising her younger children?

◆ What if Riley had to be admitted overnight?

Case 2.5 Discussion

Is Janine doing anything wrong by leaving Kyron supervising her younger children?

There is no minimum age at which children in the UK can be left on their own. Despite this, a parent can be prosecuted under the Children and Young Persons Act 1933 for wilful neglect if they leave a child unsupervised 'in a manner likely to cause unnecessary suffering or injury to health'. The National Society for the Prevention of Cruelty to Children (NSPCC, 2012) advises that:

- children under the age of about 12 are rarely mature enough to be left alone for a long period of time

- children under the age of 16 should not be left alone overnight

- babies, toddlers, and very young children should never be left alone.

Laws in the UK also do not specify how old someone needs to be to babysit. However, if the babysitter is under 16, then the parent of the children being looked after remains legally responsible for the child's safety. The NSPCC recommends that children under 16 should not be put in charge of younger children, but often it depends on the maturity of the teenager and the number and age of the younger children they are expected to look after.

What if Riley had to be admitted overnight?

Whilst it may be legal for this mother to leave Kyron babysitting for a short period of time, it is not recommended for a 14-year-old to be left alone overnight in charge of two younger children. It would be best if she asked a friend or relative to provide support during Riley's admission. If she is unable to find child care, Riley is at least safe in hospital with nursing staff whilst she goes home to provide care for her other children. Social care can provide emergency foster care for children in circumstances where parents are admitted to hospital because of their own ill-health.

Conclusion

Although not exhaustive, this chapter covers the important laws within the child protection framework and some areas which are not covered under the law, such as the minimum age for babysitting or leaving children at home alone.

References

Children Act 1989 (c.41). London: HMSO.

Children Act 2004 (c.31). London: HMSO.

Children and Young Persons Act 1933 (c.12). London, HMSO.

Children (Northern Ireland) Order 1995. London: HMSO. Available at: http://www.legislation. gov.uk/nisi/1995/755/contents/made (accessed 19 August 2013).

Civic Government (Scotland) Act 1982 (c.50 (2)).

Deater-Deckard, K., Dodge, K.A. (1997). Externalizing behavior problems and discipline revisited: nonlinear effects and variation by culture, context, and gender. *Psychological Inquiry*, **8(3)**, 161–75.

Domestic Violence, Crime and Victims Act 2004. Available at: http://www.legislation.gov.uk/ ukpga/2004/28/contents (accessed 18 August 2013).

Gershoff, E.T. (2002). Corporal punishment by parents and associated child behaviors and experiences: a meta-analytic and theoretical review. *Psychological Bulletin*, **128**(4), 539–79.

GMC (2012). *Protecting Children and Young People: The Responsibilities of All Doctors*. Available at: http://www.gmc-uk.org/Protecting_children_and_young_people___English_0414. pdf_48978248.pdf (accessed 24 September 2014).

Hayden, T. L. (1980). Classification of elective mutism. *Journal of the American Academy of Child Psychiatry*, **19**, 118–33.

Law Reform (Miscellaneous Provisions) (Northern Ireland) Order 2006. Available at: http://www. legislation.gov.uk/nisi/2006/1945/contents/made (accessed 18 August 2013).

Licensing Act 1902 (c.1 (2)). London: HMSO.

Munro, E. (2011). *The Munro Review of Child Protection: Final Report—A Child-Centred System*. London: TSO.

NSPCC (2012). *Home Alone: Your Guide to Keeping Your Child Safe*. Available at: http://www. nspcc.org.uk/help-and-advice/for-parents-and-carers/guides-for-parents/home-alone/ home-alone-pdf_wdf90656.pdf (accessed 18 August 2013).

RCN (2007). *Safeguarding Children and Young People: Every Nurse's Responsibility*. Available at: http://www.rcn.org.uk/__data/assets/pdf_file/0004/78583/004542.pdf (accessed 24 September 2014).

Scotland's Children—The Children (Scotland) Act 1995 Regulations and Guidance: Volume 1 Support and Protection for Children and Their Families. Available at: http://www.scotland.gov. uk/Publications/2004/10/20066/44708 (accessed 18 August 2013).

Steele, B.D., Brennan, P.O. (2002). A prospective survey of patients with presumed accidental ear injury presenting to a paediatric accident and emergency department. *Emergency Medicine Journal*, **19** (3), 226–8.

3

The consequences of child maltreatment and the public health perspective

Benita Morrissey

Chapter summary

Child maltreatment is a global problem that affects children in every society across the world, with far-reaching consequences. Every year an estimated 31,000 children die from child abuse worldwide (World Health Organization, 2014). Many more experience long-lasting adverse consequences. This chapter will consider the impact that child maltreatment can have on children in terms of its physical, psychological, and behavioural effects, many of which persist into adulthood. The wider cost to society of child maltreatment will also be discussed with the argument that this is a significant public health issue requiring a multidisciplinary coordinated public health approach to address it.

Case 3.1 The consequences of physical abuse and neglect

You are a paediatric doctor in the community carrying out a 'looked after child' medical assessment on three-year-old Alexander. Alexander is accompanied by his social worker, Rachel, and foster carer, Sarah. Alex has been in foster care for the last two years. He was removed from his birth parents at one year of age because of physical abuse and neglect. At that time Alexander had severe faltering growth and delayed development. Whilst in the care of his parents he had sustained a femoral fracture that was thought to be non-accidental. Alexander's mother was 20 years old at the time and had a history of depression and deliberate self-harm. Alexander's father was 24 years old. Alexander now attends a nursery three mornings a week, but Sarah is still concerned that he seems small for his age and she thinks that his development is behind that of her other children. Sarah is considering adopting Alexander and asks you if Alexander is likely to continue to experience difficulties into later childhood and adolescence.

Case 3.1 Exercise

♦ What are the possible consequences of the neglect and physical abuse that Alexander has experienced?

♦ What factors influence the effects of child maltreatment on children?

♦ Could Alexander continue to experience difficulties lasting into adolescence and beyond?

♦ What can you do for Alexander?

Case 3.1 Discussion

What are the possible consequences of the neglect and physical abuse that Alexander has experienced?

Child maltreatment can have significant physical consequences. Physical health problems, and in severe cases death, can arise directly from the injuries received, as in Alexander's case, such as cuts, bruises, burns, fractures, and haemorrhage. Abusive head trauma (shaken baby syndrome) is the most common cause of traumatic death in infants and can cause severe neurodevelopmental delay, hearing and speech problems, impaired vision, and blindness in surviving infants.

Alexander also had severe faltering growth due to neglect. During the first two years a child's brain grows rapidly, and even moderate nutritional deprivation during this period of rapid brain growth and differentiation can lead to adverse neurodevelopmental outcomes. Neglect is associated with developmental delay, particularly delays in expressive language and imaginative play.

What factors influence the effects of child maltreatment on children?

Child maltreatment can affect children differently. Some children function adequately despite being subject to significant abuse. Individual, family, and community factors can impact upon a child's vulnerability or resilience to maltreatment. Resilience is the ability of the child to resist adversity, cope with uncertainty, and recover successfully from trauma. Individual factors affecting resilience are a child's positive self-esteem, intelligence, independence, good communication skills, and sense of humour. Family factors include a close bond with at least one person, closeness with grandparents, and sibling attachment. Community factors affecting resilience include having friends, support from other adults such as teachers, and good experiences at school. The way in which abuse and neglect affect children and adolescents also depends on the age and developmental stage of the child when the maltreatment occurred, the severity, frequency, duration, and type of the maltreatment, and the relationship between the child and the perpetrator.

Could Alexander continue to experience difficulties lasting into adolescence?

Child maltreatment can have long-lasting physical effects, and several studies have reported associations between child maltreatment and ischaemic heart disease, cancer, chronic lung disease, and liver disease in adulthood (Gilbert et al., 2009) Those who have been maltreated as children are more likely to engage in smoking, drinking alcohol, and engaging in risky behaviour, which can give rise to physical health problems. (Norman et al., 2012) Child abuse is also strongly associated with obesity in later life.

What can you do for Alexander?

Early detection of health and neurodevelopmental problems is essential in children who have experienced maltreatment. Alexander should have an assessment of his development, and if delayed, he should be referred to the child development team. Any potentially reversible or treatable causes of developmental delay, such as visual or auditory impairments, need to be excluded. Basic growth parameters such as height, weight, and head circumference must be measured and marked on an appropriate growth chart. Alexander may also have missed out on other important health interventions, such as immunizations, and it is important that these are given.

Case 3.2 The consequences of emotional and sexual abuse

You are the paediatric registrar on call one afternoon when a nurse from the Paediatric Emergency Department calls you about Davina, a 14-year-old girl who has been brought in by ambulance. She disclosed to a friend at school that she had taken 17 paracetamol tablets before school that morning because she was 'feeling low'. Her friend told the form tutor, who called an ambulance.

Davina's schoolteacher Pete, who accompanies her, tells the nurse that she lives with her maternal aunt. She was previously subject to a child protection plan under the categories of sexual and emotional abuse. She has occasional contact with her mother but none with her father, who was the perpetrator of the abuse. Pete tells the nurse that they are all very worried about Davina as she has missed a lot of school recently, and there have been rumours going around the school that she has been 'cutting herself'. The nurse tells you that Davina's observations are normal.

Case 3.2 Exercise

- What do you do for Davina?

- What could be contributing to Davina's current presentation?

- What are the possible emotional and behavioural consequences of child maltreatment?

- What are the wider costs to society of child maltreatment?

Case 3.2 Discussion

What do you do for Davina?

Davina will require a full medical and psychiatric assessment and probably admission at least overnight until Child and Adolescent Mental Health Services can assess her. Her paracetamol overdose should be managed as per national guidelines. You need to take a detailed history from Davina. It will be important to see Davina on her own (but possibly accompanied by a nurse or colleague) so she has the opportunity to tell you about anything that is worrying her or has triggered this episode. A social care referral should be considered and discussed with your consultant, given the presentation and concerns from the school.

What could be contributing to Davina's current presentation?

There are many possible factors that could have contributed to Davina's current presentation, but it is likely that the emotional and sexual abuse that she experienced previously is a significant contributor.

Child maltreatment has both immediate emotional effects, including isolation, fear, and an inability to trust, and longer-lasting psychological consequences.

Depression, severe anxiety, panic attacks, and post-traumatic stress disorder are the most common mental health consequences.

Self-harm is also strongly associated with sexual abuse, although not necessarily with physical abuse and neglect. Both physical and sexual abuse are associated with a doubling of the suicide risk for young people. One British study of suicidal behaviour found that while only 4 per cent of the population had attempted suicide, 22 per cent of those who had experienced violence in the home during childhood and 26 per cent of those who had been sexually abused had done so (Meadows et al., 2011) Children who have experienced physical and sexual abuse are also much more likely to experience intimate partner violence as adults.

What are the possible educational consequences of child maltreatment?

Child maltreatment is associated with developmental delay, cognitive problems, and adverse educational outcomes. Children who have experienced child maltreatment are more likely than their peers to have poorer educational attainment and require special educational support. They are less likely to complete secondary schooling and attain a university degree. Maltreatment is also associated with being suspended or expelled from school and increased absenteeism. This is significant as persistent absenteeism is a predictor of lower employment rates and lower earnings in later life. Children who have been maltreated can have difficulties with attachments and interpersonal relationships later in life and have been found to be three times more likely to have no close friends than non-maltreated children (NSPCC, 1996).

What are the wider costs to society of child maltreatment?

In addition to the costs to the child, there is an association between child maltreatment and criminal behaviour. The proportion of children and young people in custody who have experienced maltreatment is over twice that in the population as a whole. Whilst there is no evidence that maltreatment causes youth offending, it is one of the factors contributing to children and young people following pathways that make offending more likely. Abused and neglected children are also at increased risk of displaying aggressive behaviour to others. These findings have led to concerns about the 'cycle of violence', where children who have experienced maltreatment or witnessed violence between their parents and caregivers are more likely to subject their children to maltreatment.

Individuals who have histories of childhood abuse and neglect can experience long-lasting economic consequences. Child maltreatment has effects on education, employment, occupation, earnings, and assets, which appear to affect women more strongly than men (Currie and Widom, 2011).

Although much attention has been paid to detection of child maltreatment and the protection of children from further harm, there also needs to be a focus on prevention. More research is required to learn what works in prevention at an individual and policy level, and how to promote resilience in children and families. Communities need to develop evidence-based strategies and programmes that prevent child maltreatment both to alleviate childhood suffering and to prevent the later life and societal problems that occur as a consequence.

Conclusion

Child maltreatment is a major public health problem. It has significant long-lasting consequences for the individual children who experience it, and also carries a significant burden for society as a whole. In the USA, it is estimated that child maltreatment costs $124 billion in direct costs each year, with each case costing society around $210,000. There are also indirect economic costs from increased use of the healthcare system, youth offending, mental health problems, and substance abuse. There have been no studies of the economic costs of child maltreatment in the UK. Any estimates have been based on extrapolations from US figures. It is likely that the economic cost of child maltreatment runs into billions of pounds, but whatever the figure, it is a cost that we cannot afford.

References

Currie, J. and Widom, C.S. (2011). long-term consequences of child abuse and neglect on adult economic well-being. *Child Maltreatment*, **15** (2), 111–20.

Gilbert, R., Widom, C.S., Browne, K., Fergusson, D., Webb, E., Janson, S. (2009). Burden and consequences of child maltreatment in high-income countries. *Lancet*, **373**(9657), 68–81.

Meadows, P., Tunstill, J., George, A., Dhudwar, A., Kurtz, A. (2011). *The Costs and Consequences of Child Maltreatment: Literature Review for the NSPCC*. London:NSPCC.

NSPCC (1996). National Commission of Inquiry into the Prevention of Child Abuse. Childhood Matters, Vols 1 and 2. London: NSPCC.

Norman, R.E., Byambaa, M., De, R., Butchart, A., Scott, J., Vos, T. (2012). The long-term health consequences of child physical abuse, emotional abuse, and neglect: a systematic review and meta-analysis. *PloS Medicine*, **9**(11), e1001349. Available at: http://www.ploscollections.org/article/info%3Adoi%2F10.1371%2Fjournal.pmed.1001349 (accessed 25 September 2014).

World Health Organization (2014). *Child Maltreatment*. Available at: http://www.who.int/mediacentre/factsheets/fs150/en/ (accessed 25 September 2014).

4

Challenges to professionals working in child protection

Kerry Robinson and Maryam Hyrapetian

Chapter summary

Disciplinary action by the General Medical Council (GMC) against paediatricians such as David Southall and Roy Meadow, and how this has resulted in discouraging paediatricians from working in the field of child protection, is discussed in this chapter. The media vilification of paediatricians in high-profile cases and its psychological impact on doctors dealing with child protection cases is discussed.

Introduction to challenges to professionals working in child protection

Paediatricians must be able to undertake child protection work competently and confidently. In 2012 the GMC published revised guidance explicitly outlining the duties of doctors to report possible child abuse and neglect. The GMC aims to provide reassurance that where concerns are honestly held and reasonable, doctors are able to use their professional judgment, clearly justifying their decisions and actions with the aim of removing the threat of complaints or disciplinary action.

High-profile cases and the impact of media coverage in child protection

High-profile cases in which paediatricians have been maligned in the press provoke a great deal of anxiety in clinicians undertaking child protection work.

There is criticism for failing to recognize child abuse, and there is also criticism for over-diagnosis (Cass, 2014). Paediatricians acting as expert witnesses have been accused of mistaken 'allegations', as in the cases of Sir Roy Meadow and Professor David Southall.

Both Meadow and Southall were influential and highly regarded paediatricians of their generation, specifically within the field of child protection. Meadow was knighted in 1998 for his contributions to child welfare and Southall received an OBE for his work as founder of the charity Maternity and Childhealth Advocacy International. Even though their work has potentially saved many children from unnecessary suffering, their careers have become blighted by controversy, scepticism, and criticism of their once highly regarded expert views.

Cases like these undermine public confidence in paediatricians and leaves them in the position of 'damned if you do, damned if you don't' when confronted with potential child abuse cases (Kmietowicz, 2004).

Sir Roy Meadow

Sir Roy Meadow first came to prominence in 1977 after publishing a paper in *The Lancet* on a condition he named Munchausen syndrome by proxy. He postulated that carers induce real or apparent symptoms of disease in children in order to gain attention from medical professionals. Meadow suggested that sudden infant death syndrome and Munchausen syndrome by proxy were closely related, and this theory led him to become influential. However, there was severe criticism of his testimonies at the court trials of three women: Sally Clark, Angela Cannings, and Donna Anthony. These women were convicted of murdering their children, with Meadow's theories being used as support for their convictions, but they were later exonerated by the Court of Appeal after serving time in prison. This had damning implications for Meadow's career, leading to accusations against him of inventing a 'theory without science'.

In 2005 Meadow appeared before a GMC Fitness to Practise Panel where it was ruled that his evidence in the Sally Clark case, including the statistical calculation he had given on the odds of two cot deaths within one family, was misleading. He was found guilty of serious professional misconduct and his name was removed from the general medical register.

The following month Meadow launched an appeal against the ruling. A High Court judge ruled against the decision to strike him from the medical register; the criticism from the GMC was deemed appropriate but his actions could not properly be regarded as 'serious professional misconduct'. It was concluded that although Meadow was guilty of some professional misconduct, it did not equate to serious misconduct.

Concern was expressed by the Society of Expert Witnesses that this case would cause many professionals to reconsider whether to stand as expert witnesses. The law was then changed so that no person could be convicted on the basis of expert testimony alone.

Professor David Southall

Professor David Southall also became viewed as a leading expert on Munchausen syndrome by proxy. From 1986 to 1994 he led a research project using covert video surveillance to investigate apparent life-threatening events. His group demonstrated that some parents were causing suffocation by deliberate airway obstruction. In 1997 the project became the focus of multiple complaints from parents and extensive press coverage criticized the methods and ethics of the research. This culminated in GMC disciplinary action against Southall.

Southall was also at the centre of controversy following a study in which he pioneered continuous negative extrathoracic pressure for premature babies. Southall and his colleagues were accused of experimenting without parental consent, with some parents also suggesting that the treatment could be linked to subsequent death or severe brain damage. David Southall was suspended by his employers in 1999, but was cleared of any wrongdoing and reinstated in 2001.

In 2004 Southall provoked further controversy regarding the Sally Clark case. After watching a television interview with her husband Steve Clark, Southall suggested to police that Steve Clark, rather than his convicted wife, might have been guilty of killing their sons. A High Court judge declared that Southall's theory was seriously flawed, and the GMC Panel subsequently found him guilty of serious professional misconduct, banning him from undertaking child protection work for four years.

Southall finally emerged from multiple GMC disciplinary hearings in 2012 with full GMC licence to practice. Given his background and the fact he had lost his NHS job (along with his pension and merit award), returning to work was not straightforward.

Despite the controversy and scepticism surrounding the careers of these two high-profile paediatricians, their work has undoubtedly educated the medical profession and public about Munchausen syndrome by proxy, which is now known as *fabricated and induced illness* (see Chapter 10).

Case 4.1 Complex epilepsy

A six-year-old boy, Michael, was diagnosed with absence seizures when he was three and a half years old. He was investigated with two electroencephalographs

(EEGs), both of which were normal. Hyperventilation was attempted, but compliance was difficult. This was considered acceptable due to his age. A diagnosis was made on a convincing history and he was initially treated with ethosuximide.

Prescribed medications were primarily administered by his mother or under her control and direction. The ethosuximide had no effect on his seizures; his mother continued to report up to 20 events per day. School reports were difficult to obtain accurately—the teacher said that in a class of 30 children she found it really difficult to watch Michael all the time. The school did not have enough staff for someone to stay with Michael all day. They did report that his performance was lagging behind that of other children his age.

In view of this, his medication was changed, but his 'fits' deteriorated. There was never conclusive proof of epilepsy despite repeated consultations and investigations, and no one other than his mother ever witnessed him having a seizure.

Case 4.1 Exercise

◆ What concerns you so far about this story?

◆ Who could you turn to for help?

◆ What other agencies would you involve?

Case 4.1 Discussion

What concerns you so far about this story?

There are a number of concerning features of fabricated and induced illness:

◆ Inconclusive proof of a diagnosis of epilepsy despite repeated consultations and investigations.

◆ 'Seizures' were never witnessed by anybody else, and yet his mother explains that despite trials of different medications over a period of time his 'fits' allegedly deteriorated.

◆ Prescribed medications were primarily administered by his mother or under her control and direction.

Who could you turn to for help?

Support for paediatricians Cases such as these are stressful and carrying the responsibility alone is very hard. Networks and support are invaluable and can make safeguarding work very rewarding (Hall, 2003).

You could discuss this case with others:

♦ The team in the hospital—other consultant colleagues, the named doctor for child safeguarding in the trust, the area designated doctor for safeguarding, the liaison health visitor, or the designated nurse for safeguarding.

♦ The case could be taken to supervision—it is good practice for the lead clinician for child safeguarding in a trust to be linked into a supervision network where cases such as this are discussed to obtain other perspectives.

What other agencies would you involve?

Multidisciplinary working Information sharing is vital—you may have only one piece of the jigsaw. Multidisciplinary working is an essential part of safeguarding children. Early involvement of different agencies facilitates a collaborative approach to information gathering, discussion and decision-making.

♦ It would be a good idea to contact the general practitioner. The GP can share information about the mother as long as it is in the best interests of the child. This could give good insight into illness-seeking behaviour and the mother's mental health. The GP may also have information about attendances at other hospitals.

♦ The school may have important information—the school nurse may be helpful or you can contact the child's teacher. Always keep in mind sharing of information across professional boundaries—it can be done if it is in the best interests of the child (information sharing is covered in Chapter 2, Case 2.4).

♦ A professionals meeting, where concerned professionals meet to share information, could be held. The mother and child are not invited to attend. An expert in the area of factitious or induced illness could be asked to review the history.

♦ Discuss this case with social care. It may not meet their threshold for investigation but they can provide guidance.

While multi-agency working is pivotal to the successful management of child maltreatment cases, it can also bring additional challenges. It involves not just information sharing but understanding roles and responsibilities across professional boundaries and developing trust between practitioners.

> ## Case 4.1 Exercise continued
>
> ◆ What would you say to Michael's mother?
>
> ◆ When would you raise the issue that you think she may be causing harm to Michael?

Case 4.1 continued

It was discovered later that Michael's mother had obtained quantities of the pre-scribed medication which were far in excess of his requirements. Toxic effects went on to cause chronic poor health for Michael. He was eventually unable to attend school and required naso-gastric administration of feed and drugs.

At the age of seven years Michael died following severe aspiration pneumonia. This was thought to be secondary to medication being administered via a dis-lodged nasogastric tube that had become positioned in his trachea. It later tran-spired that his mother had re-sited the nasogastric tube herself without alerting community nursing teams, the GP, or the hospital.

Communicating concerns

Although both Royal College of Paediatrics and Child Health (RCPCH) and GMC guidance is to be open and honest with parents, it is particularly difficult in cases of suspected factitious or induced illness. The language used to com-municate concerns to the mother is essential to contain the situation. It is useful to rehearse this with someone who has done it before.

Once concerns of possible child maltreatment are communicated, the shift in the normal collaborative partnership between doctors and parents changes. In an article about the difficulties of child protection work in the climate of recent years, Payne (2008) highlights that however calmly and impartially concerns are expressed to parents, their response is inevitably that they are accused of abusing their child.

The recommendations of the Laming Report (2003) make it very clear that where there are concerns about deliberate harm these must be shared and recorded in the child's medical record.

Training for doctors

Effective child protection is only possible if there is adequate training of prac-titioners in the field, alongside experienced clinical leadership. A survey by

Zalkin et al. (2011) found that trainees rated training in child protection as poorer than other areas of paediatrics, with 33 per cent feeling that they would not be able to undertake this work competently and confidently as consultants. Over 50 per cent said that they would be more likely to undertake this work in the future if support and training were improved. This supports the results of an RCPCH survey in 2007. This plea echoes Lord Laming's recommendation that expert advice and regular training updates should be readily available for all grades of doctor.

Despite the development of child protection training by the RCPCH, it is clear that training for all grades needs to be improved with clear, structured, mandatory, and accessible programmes starting at undergraduate level and continuing indefinitely.

Conclusion

Child protection will always be a rewarding, but difficult and stressful, area of paediatric practice. Paediatricians must be able to engage in the important task of protecting children without feeling that they are putting their careers and their own families at risk. It is extremely important that there is a culture where specialists no longer feel so constrained by the burden of certainty that suspicions are not shared.

It is also important that the profile of child protection is raised in the public domain and in the correct format to increase knowledge and understanding. Campaigns such as 'Full Stop' and 'The Underwear Rule' by the National Society for the Prevention of Cruelty to Children go some way towards addressing this. Such moves will work towards developing and maintaining relationships between paediatricians and parents when child abuse is suspected.

References

Cass, H. (2014). Child protection: a blend of art and science. *Archives of Disease in Childhood*, **99** (2), 101–2.

GMC (2012). *Protecting Children and Young People: The Responsibilities of All Doctors*. Available at: http://www.gmc-uk.org/guidance/ethical_guidance/13257.asp (accessed 27 September 2014).

Hall, D. (2003). Protecting children, supporting professionals. *Archives of Disease in Childhood*, 88(7), 557–9.

Kmietowicz, Z. (2004). Complaints against doctors in child protection work have increased fivefold. *British Medical Journal*, **328**(7440), 601.

Laming Report (2003). *The Victoria Climbié Inquiry*. Available at: http://www.official-documents.gov.uk/document/cm57/5730/5730.pdf (accessed 10 September 2014).

Payne, H. (2008). The jigsaw of child protection. *Journal of the Royal Society of Medicine*, **101**(2), 93–4.

Zalkin, M.D., Fertleman, C., Hodes, D. (2011). Paediatric registrar's views on current child protection training and willingness to undertake child protection work in the current climate: what needs to be done? *Archives of Disease in Childhood*, **96**(Suppl 1), A97. Available at: http://adc.bmj.com/content/96/Suppl_1/A97.1.abstract (accessed 27 September 2014).

5

Definitions and types of abuse

Laura Haynes and Gayle Hann

Chapter summary

This chapter will cover the risk factors and indicators of different types of abuse. The types and definitions of physical, emotional, and sexual abuse will be described in addition to neglect.

Defining child abuse

The term 'child abuse' refers to maltreatment of a child causing significant harm. 'Harm' is defined as 'ill-treatment' or 'the impairment of health or development' of the child. 'Ill-treatment' includes sexual abuse and forms of ill-treatment which are not physical (Children Act 1989). Abuse and neglect can occur as a direct result of the actions of others, or as an indirect result of a person failing to act in order to prevent harm. Harm to a child can be inflicted in a number of ways, and four broad classifications of abuse are used: physical, sexual, emotional, and neglect.

The well-being and health of all children is dependent on parents and carers; for this reason children are more vulnerable to maltreatment than most adults, and therefore are more likely to be abused or neglected. Abuse and neglect occur in all social classes, all cultures, and all ethnicities; however, there are certain factors which make some children more vulnerable than others (see Box 5.1). These factors may affect the child, the family, or society as a whole.

Physical abuse

Physical abuse includes any actions which inflict bodily harm to a child; this can be via forceful or violent acts such as hitting, biting, burning, suffocating, or shaking; or non-violent acts such as poisoning or deliberately inducing or fabricating illness.

Box 5.1 Risk factors for abuse and neglect

Child

◆ Serious illness

◆ Premature birth/low birth weight

◆ Disability (physical/cognitive/emotional)

◆ Age (less than two years, and adolescent)

◆ Behavioural problems (aggression/attention deficits)

◆ Difficult temperament

Family

◆ Parental mental health problems

◆ Parental drug or alcohol abuse

◆ Social isolation

◆ Domestic violence/parental conflict

◆ Single parenthood

◆ Many children

◆ Poor interactions between parent and child

Environmental

◆ Homelessness

◆ Parental unemployment

◆ Poor/unsuitable housing

◆ High crime rate in local area

◆ Low socio-economic status

◆ Insufficient social support

This list is not exhaustive.

Case 5.1 Physical abuse in a six-month-old child

You are called to see a six-month-old girl, Sarah, with her mother, Monica, who was worried that Sarah had injured her head after rolling off a bed at home. She reports that the previous night she had placed Sarah in the middle of the bed when she heard her sons arguing and had left the room to intervene. She returned to the bedroom when she heard Sarah crying, and found her lying on her back on the floor. At first she states that Sarah was left alone in the room, but later admits that her boyfriend was asleep in the bed at the time. Monica says that she didn't bring Sarah to hospital that evening as she thought that she was fine, but today was worried because she was unsettled and had developed a bruise.

You take a full history and learn that Sarah is otherwise well with no significant medical history. She lives with Monica and Monica's boyfriend, David, who moved in four months ago, and two older brothers, Darren and James.

You examine Sarah, who is alert and crying, and notice a 2 cm circular bruise under her right eye and multiple 1 cm oval bruises on the sides of her back. Monica provides Sarah's red book which shows that all immunizations are up to date and that she has followed the 25th centile for height and weight since birth.

You are concerned about Sarah and check to see whether she or her brothers have a child protection plan in place, and phone social care for any further information. The family are not previously known to social care.

Case 5.1 Exercise

♦ What are your concerns?

♦ Are there any concerning features in the history?

♦ Are there any concerning features in examination findings?

Case 5.1 Discussion

What are your concerns?

The possibility of physical abuse must be considered. Bruising in relatively immobile young children should not be ignored.

Are there any concerning features in the history?

♦ Delay in presentation: Sarah was brought over 12 hours after the incident.

♦ The explanation given does not fit with injury seen: mother states the baby rolled off the bed onto the floor and was found on her back, yet the bruise is underneath her eye.

♦ Elements of history changed or omitted: mother first said that Sarah was left alone before admitting that her boyfriend was with her.

◆ Injury in an infant who is not independently mobile: although at six months it is possible that Sarah did roll off the bed by herself, it does not explain her facial bruise or the bruises on her trunk. Non-accidental injury should be considered.

Are there any concerning features in examination findings?

◆ Sarah has a bruise underneath her eye and multiple small bruises on her trunk which could be fingertip bruising; both raise concerns of abuse (see Box 5.2).

Box 5.2   Concerning features in physical abuse

Any physical injury where explanation is unsuitable or absent

Bruising

◆ Bruising in children who are not independently mobile

◆ Multiple bruising or bruises in clusters

◆ Bruises that are away from bony prominences

◆ Bruises to face, eyes, ears, trunk, arms, buttocks, and hands

◆ Bruises that carry the imprint of a hand, ligature, or implement

Bites, lacerations, abrasions, and scars

◆ Report/appearance of a human bite mark

◆ Lacerations, abrasions, or scars with an unsuitable explanation, especially if multiple, symmetrical, and on areas usually covered by clothing or on the face

◆ Abrasions and scars on neck/ankles or wrists that look like ligature marks

Burns and scalds

◆ Burns or scalds on an area which would not be expected to come into contact with a hot object accidentally

◆ Burns indicating forced immersion: scalds in glove or stocking distribution, to buttocks or perineum, or with sharp delineated borders

Fractures

◆ Fractures of different ages

◆ History of multiple fractures in the absence of predisposing conditions (osteogenesis imperfecta) or a suitable explanation

◆ Child less than three years old

Head injury

- ◆ Intracranial injury
- ◆ Child less than three years old
- ◆ Retinal haemorrhages
- ◆ Multiple subdural haemorrhages

Data from NICE, (2009)

Sexual abuse

Sexual abuse includes any actions which force or coerce a child into participating in or observing sexual practices. A more detailed definition can be found in Chapter 7, Sexual abuse.

Case 5.2 Sexual abuse

A 14-year-old girl, Zoe, has come alone to see you, her GP. Zoe reluctantly tells you that she is worried because she has recently had some abnormal vaginal discharge. She admits that she has been sexually active with her boyfriend, Sean, for about a year, and that they don't always use condoms. Zoe is worried that her mother will find out as none of her family know about Sean and would not approve. When you ask why her family would not approve, Zoe reveals that he is older, 24 years old, and that he has been her gymnastics coach for four years. Zoe is adamant that her family cannot find out, and that the age gap doesn't matter because she and Sean love each other.

Case 5.2 Exercise

- ◆ What are your concerns?
- ◆ What are the concerning features in the history?

Case 5.2 Discussion

What are your concerns?

Zoe is being sexually abused; she is a 14-year-old girl who has been sexually active for a year with a 24-year-old man.

What are the concerning features in the history?

◆ She has disclosed being sexually active with an adult in a position of responsibility

◆ She has genital symptoms: abnormal vaginal discharge (see Box 5.3).

Box 5.3 Concerning features that may indicate sexual abuse

◆ Allegation or disclosure of sexual abuse

◆ Sexual activity or pregnancy in a young person less than 17 years old

◆ Sexually transmitted infection

◆ Anogenital injury with unsuitable explanation

◆ Vaginal bleeding without medical explanation or history of trauma

◆ Unexplained rectal bleeding (exclude causes such as anal fissure, inflammatory bowel disease, or infective diarrhoea)

◆ Vaginal discharge or vulvovaginitis (common, but consider abuse if recurrent or resistant to treatment)

◆ Soiling or enuresis

◆ Foreign body in vagina or anus

◆ Behavioural change including low mood, self-harm, poor school performance, sexualized behaviours, anxiety, and withdrawal

Data from NICE, (2013).

Emotional abuse

Emotional abuse includes any behaviours or interactions towards a child which cause emotional distress that is significant enough to be detrimental to the child's emotional development and well-being. An in-depth definition is given in Chapter 8.

Emotional abuse is very difficult to identify, as there is no definitive test or sign (see Chapter 8 for worrying signs). However, it should be considered in all children who have suffered any other form of abuse or neglect, as it is likely that the abuse suffered will have had an impact on the emotional well-being of the child.

Neglect

Neglect is defined as a failure of a parent or carer to meet the basic physical and emotional needs of a child, significant enough to negatively impact the development or health of the child (see Box 5.4 for concerning features of neglect).

> **Box 5.4** Concerning features suggesting neglect
> - Failure to attend routine child health appointments (e.g. immunizations), or to seek medical advice when necessary, or to administer prescribed medication
> - Poor school attendance or achievement
> - Failure to thrive or faltering growth
> - Inappropriate, dirty, or ill-fitting clothing
> - Poor hygiene: dirty or smelly, persistent infestations (e.g. head lice or scabies)
> - Frequent accidents as a result of poor supervision or unsafe home
> - Abandonment: parent or carer leaves the child without adult supervision or carer
>
> Adapted from RCPCH, (2013).

Case 5.3 Emotional abuse and neglect

You are called to see James, a seven-year-old boy, who attends with a school teacher as he had been limping during a sports lesson. James is complaining of pain in his right great toe, and when you examine him you notice that he has an itchy rash all over his body and an infected in-growing toenail on his right great toe. He reports that he has had the rash for three months and that others in his family have the same rash. You suspect that the rash is caused by scabies (see Figures 5.1 and 5.2).

Jamie looks small for his age and is unkempt, with dirty hair and clothing and holes in his shoes. His weight is below the 0.4th centile on a growth chart and his height is on the 9th centile. A nurse finds you and tells you that when she told James she had called his mother, he said that he didn't think she would come as she doesn't like him because he is a nuisance. When Jamie's mother arrives, you notice that she expresses little concern over the situation and makes no attempt to comfort him.

You discover that Jamie does not have a child protection plan, but the family are known to social care as they were assessed a year ago when his mother attended the emergency department after taking a deliberate overdose and was suffering from severe depression.

> **Case 5.3 Exercise**
> - What are your concerns?
> - What are the concerning features in the history?

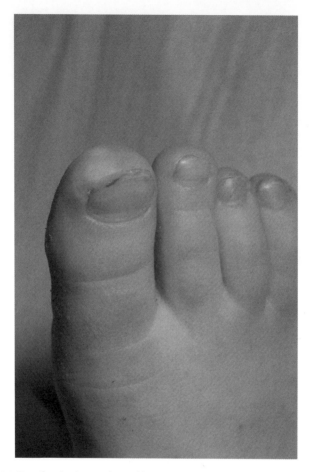

Figure 5.1 Poor foot hygiene with roughly cut nails and blistered great toe from badly fitting shoes (see also colour plate section).

Case 5.3 Discussion

What are your concerns?

Jamie is being neglected. He has a skin rash that has been present for three months for which his mother has not sought medical advice or treatment. He is also underweight, his clothes are in poor condition, and he has poor hygiene.

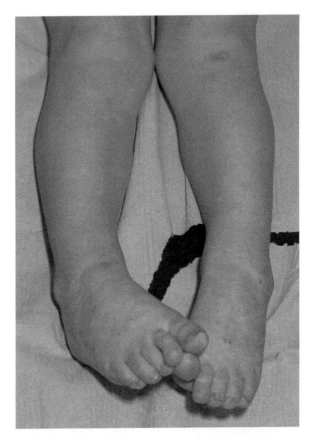

Figure 5.2 Unkempt with multiple scabbed lesions from scabies (see also colour plate section).

It is also possible that he is being emotionally abused, suggested by Jamie's comments about his mother's opinion of him, and her indifferent attitude towards him.

What are the concerning features in the history?

◆ Faltering growth

◆ Poor personal hygiene

◆ Dirty clothing and broken shoes.

Conclusion

In summary, it is important to identify the concerning features in history and examination in any case of suspected abuse or neglect. Management of suspected abuse and neglect is discussed in later chapters.

References

Children Act 1989. Available at: http://www.legislation.gov.uk/ukpga/1989/41/contents. (accessed 31 January 2014).

NICE (National Institute of Clinical Excellence). (2009). *When to Suspect Child Maltreatment*. Available at: http://www.nice.org.uk/CG89 (accessed 31 January 2014).

RCPCH (Royal College of Paediatrics and Child Health). (2013). *The Child Protection Companion*. Available at: http://www.rcpch.ac.uk/child-protection-companion (accessed 31 January 2014).

6

Physical abuse

Hannah Jacob

Chapter summary

This chapter discusses physical abuse, defined as any non-accidental injury inflicted on a child. Through a series of vignettes, it identifies key features in the history and examination that suggest an injury is non-accidental in nature. Cases ranging from bruising and fractures to burns and head injury are included. In each example, the discussion which follows highlights important aspects of early management including the investigations to consider.

Case 6.1 Non-accidental head injury

You are called to the Emergency Department as two-month-old Freddy arrives. He is with his aunt Angela who called an ambulance when his eyes rolled back and all four limbs began shaking. This lasted for approximately six minutes and terminated shortly after the ambulance crew arrived. Freddy's temperature was 37.1°C. He is now sleepy, and is maintaining his airway with an oxygen mask applied.

Your colleagues are stabilizing Freddy while you speak to Angela to get more information. Freddy has drunk 20 ml of milk today, has vomited twice, and had dry nappies. He has no fever or rash but has been unsettled. Angela explains that Freddy has colic and wakes up every two hours overnight. Her sister Ruth 'is at the end of her tether', so Angela has been looking after Freddy today.

Case 6.1 Exercise

- Which features of the history and examination make non-accidental head injury more likely?

- How does shaking cause injury to the infant brain?

- What is the prognosis if this head injury is non-accidental?

Case 6.1 Discussion

Which features of the history and examination make non-accidental head injury more likely?

Poor feeding, vomiting, and irritability are all features of non-accidental head injury. Seizures are reported in approximately half of cases (Bechtel et al., 2004) and children may present with apnoea, respiratory distress, and hypothermia. However, many of these features are non-specific and may occur in children who are unwell for other reasons. A thorough history is essential to identify the likely cause.

It is important that you keep an open mind about the cause of a child's presentation and treat other possible causes such as infection. The history in this case is concerning. Freddy's colic means long periods of crying which, with interrupted sleep, puts him at higher risk of physical abuse. Parents or carers may shake a baby in a moment of frustration, causing brain injury.

Retinal haemorrhages (flame-shaped collections of blood from burst retinal blood vessels) are seen in up to 90 per cent of babies with non-accidental head injury. Unlike retinal haemorrhages due to other causes, these are typically numerous, involve multiple retinal layers, and spread as far as the ora serrata (near the lens) (Bechtel et al., 2004). Neither seizures nor cardiopulmonary resuscitation result in retinal haemorrhages in children.

With no history of high-impact trauma (such as a traffic accident), a depressed or basal skull fracture is highly suggestive of physical abuse.

How does shaking cause injury?

Injury is produced by shaking and the sudden deceleration of the head at the end of the shaking arc. There may also be impact, for example if the head is banged against a wall. Shaking can cause:

- tearing of bridging veins between the brain's surface and the superior sagittal sinus, causing subdural haematoma or subarachnoid haemorrhage

- movement of the brain tissue with subsequent swelling and reduction of blood supply due to vascular compression resulting in temporary apnoea, causing hypoxia.

The infant brain contains approximately 25 per cent more water and less myelin than the brain of an older child and thus is more susceptible to the effects of trauma.

What is the prognosis if this head injury is non-accidental?

The early mortality rate for non-accidental head injury is around 15–25 per cent with an 80–90 per cent chance of learning or physical disability in survivors.

Non-accidental head injury is the most common cause of death and long-term morbidity from physical abuse (Bechtel et al., 2004).

Case summary

Children with non-accidental head injury can present with a range of symptoms and signs that may mimic other causes. Effective resuscitation is vital regardless of aetiology. Younger children and those with challenging behaviour, such as excessive crying, are at higher risk.

Case 6.2 Bites

Four-year-old Lisa is attending the nurse-led clinic at her GP surgery for her pre-school immunizations with her father. The nurse notices a circular mark on the inside of her forearm which looks like a bite mark (see Figure 6.1). The nurse asks how it happened, but Lisa is interrupted by her father who says that it must have been her two-year-old brother who is teething. You are the GP who is approached by the nurse for advice.

Case 6.2 Exercise

◆ Are there any features of this history that are worrying?

◆ What is the significance of this injury?

◆ What should you do?

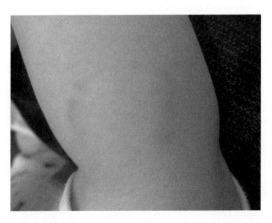

Figure 6.1 Bite to Lisa's forearm as seen at the GP surgery (see also colour plate section).

Case 6.2 Discussion

Are there any features of this history that are worrying?

It is concerning that Lisa's father interrupts her explanation. Where physical abuse is suspected, it is imperative that the child is given the opportunity to explain their injuries.

Attributing injuries to siblings is worrying (see Chapter 2, Case 2.1) and a detailed understanding of what happened is needed. It is difficult for a toddler to bite the inside of his older sister's arm. The size of the mark and individual tooth marks will help to identify whether this is a child or adult bite mark.

What is the significance of this injury?

If this is an adult human bite mark, it is a worrying sign of severe physical abuse. Marks left by a bite can be measured, photographed, and compared with dental impressions of household members (Hinchcliffe, 2011). Swabs can be taken to obtain saliva for DNA analysis.

What should you do?

You should take a thorough history from Lisa and her father, including speaking to Lisa on her own. You should examine Lisa fully to look for other injuries. You will need to make a referral to social care who will inform the police.

The safety of Lisa and her brother is paramount, and it must be decided where the children should be cared for while Lisa's injury is investigated.

Case summary

Adult bite marks are highly specific for non-accidental injury and need full and prompt investigation. Police photographs are essential as marks fade within days. It is essential to ensure the safety of siblings when planning management of a child who has potentially suffered physical abuse.

Case 6.3 Burns

Three-year-old Pablo and his mother are attending the Emergency Department because he has a rash around his buttocks. His mother says that she noticed it this morning. Pablo is visibly pained and is standing up; he says nothing when you greet him.

On examination, you notice that Pablo has an area of broken skin covering both buttocks, with unaffected skin centrally. The area looks dry and is beginning to heal from the edges. It is tender and looks like a burn.

When you question the mother further, she says that perhaps the rash has actually been there for a few days and might be a reaction to urine as Pablo is being potty trained. She states categorically that it is not a burn.

Case 6.3 Exercise

♦ What are the worrying features of this history?

♦ How do you explain the distribution of the burns?

♦ Which other body areas are more commonly affected in burns due to physical abuse?

♦ What would you do now?

Case 6.3 Discussion

What are the worrying features of this history?

Pablo's mother is changing her story about the lesions, initially saying that she noticed them that morning and then suggesting that they have been there for a few days. Inconsistencies in the history, either from an individual or between different people, are concerning.

Delayed presentation, as in this case, is more common with non-accidental injuries.

How do you explain the distribution of the burns?

The distribution, with central sparing, is typical of deliberate scalding by immersion in hot water. The centre of the buttocks may be spared because they are pressed against the colder base of the bath. This is sometimes seen during potty training when a child may be punished for wetting or soiling.

Which other body areas are commonly affected in burns due to physical abuse?

Non-accidental burns typically involve the face, head, hands, feet, and legs as well as the buttocks or genitals. Burns involving the dorsum of the hands are worrying as accidental hand burns, for example from touching a radiator, usually affect the palms.

Other common sites of immersion burns are feet and ankle burns (sock distribution) with a clear tidemark, unlike accidental scalds which leave irregular marks from splashes (Maguire et al., 2008)

Children's skin burns more easily than that of adults, particularly at high temperatures. Dry contact burns, for example from hair straighteners, should result in a reflex withdrawal and thus minor burns. Therefore any deep contact burns require explanation.

What would you do now?

You should give Pablo analgesia and dress his burns. You may have to refer him to the specialist burns unit.

A full history is needed from Pablo and his mother, and he should be examined for other features of physical abuse and infection. The infection risk is very high, particularly in the groin and anal region. Burns and any other injuries should be documented fully on body maps and photographed. You need to discuss Pablo with a senior paediatric colleague, either the named doctor for child protection or the on-call consultant. You should urgently refer him to social care and make sure that the police are involved.

Case summary

History and examination are key in distinguishing between deliberate and accidental scalds or burns. Children may need resuscitating. Adequate analgesia is essential and is often forgotten.

Case 6.4 Bruises

You see Luke, aged two years, in the Emergency Department with his mother. He has had a runny nose for three days and today is coughing more and feels hot. You notice bruises to the chest (see Figure 6.2) for which his mother has no explanation other than that he is active and 'always climbing and falling off things'. Examination otherwise reveals a red throat, coryza, and a temperature of 38.4°C.

Case 6.4 Exercise

- What are your concerns?

- Can you age the bruises?

- How should you investigate further?

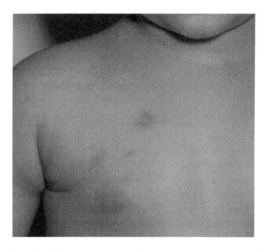

Figure 6.2 Bruises to Luke's chest as seen in the Emergency Department (see also colour plate section).

Case 6.4 Discussion

What are your concerns?

Accidental bruising is very common in a child of Luke's age, with most toddlers having at least one bruise at any time. However, you should be worried by this site. Accidental bruises typically occur over bony prominences, mostly on the front of the body such as knees and shins. Non-accidental bruises are most commonly seen on the head, neck, buttocks, and back (Maguire and Mann, 2013). These areas are more protected from falls and knocks, and so are harder to injure accidentally.

Other worrying features are multiple bruises in one area, linear bruises, or bruises with an imprint suggesting that an implement was used.

It is possible that Luke's bruises happened accidentally. A detailed history is essential to help establish the mechanism of injury.

Can you age the bruises?

It is impossible to age bruises accurately and you should not attempt to do so, either verbally or in documentation, as it cannot be done with sufficient accuracy to be reliable medico-legally (Maguire and Mann, 2013). The colour of a bruise is affected by skin colour, force and depth of the injury, and the site of the bruise, as well as your ability to detect the colour yellow, which declines with age.

How should you investigate further?

You must establish that the bruising does not have an alternative explanation such as a clotting disorder. During first-line investigations you should include a full blood count, blood film, and coagulation screen. Factor VIII, factor IX, and von Willebrand factor activity can be useful as they can prolong activated partial thromboplastin time if reduced.

In a younger child, it may be appropriate for you to carry out a skeletal survey and ophthalmic examination.

Case summary

Bruises are common in mobile infants and children. Distribution, surrounding injury, and history are useful in identifying non-accidental injury. Other causes of bruising must be ruled out.

Case 6.5 Fracture

Ama, aged four months, is brought to the hospital by her father. He reports that Ama cried when he changed her nappy and again when he dressed her. He says that she has not moved her left leg since he returned from work. She has not fallen or been injured to his knowledge.

Ama is crying and screams when you attempt to undress her. You notice swelling of her left knee. Examination is otherwise unremarkable. An x-ray shows a metaphyseal fracture of the proximal tibia.

Case 6.5 Exercise

♦ What are your concerns?

♦ What would you do?

♦ What further investigations does Ama need?

Case 6.5 Discussion

What are your concerns?

Ama has an unexplained fracture. Fractures in non-mobile infants are worrying because young infants do not usually move about enough to injure themselves like this.

Metaphyseal fractures are highly specific for non-accidental injury. These are transverse fractures caused by a shearing force across the cartilaginous growth plate. This does not occur in falling and is typically caused by pulling a child hard by the limb or shaking the torso while the limbs wave about.

What would you do?

Ama needs analgesia. You will need to discuss her with the orthopaedic team locally to ensure that her fracture is treated appropriately.

You need a detailed history from Ama's father, including any trauma and details of who has looked after her over the previous few weeks. It is important to establish whether there are other children living at home who may also be at risk.

You need to discuss Ama's case with a senior paediatrician and refer to social care. Ama needs to be kept safe while further investigations are carried out, and thus may require admission.

What further investigations does Ama need?

You may need to carry out a skeletal survey to look for other fractures. This is a series of radiographs of different parts of the body specifically aimed at detecting fractures. High-quality images are essential to enable identification and assessment of other fractures. The Royal College of Radiologists and the Royal College of Paediatrics and Child Health have produced a joint guideline (RCR/RCPCH, 2008). Ama will need analgesia prior to the skeletal survey.

Ama will need an eye examination by an ophthalmologist to look for retinal haemorrhages (see Case 6.1). She also needs blood tests for baseline bone chemistry (calcium, phosphate, and vitamin D). Other investigations may be appropriate depending on the outcome of these tests.

Case summary

Fractures in non-mobile infants are always concerning. A detailed history of any trauma is essential to establish the possible mechanism of injury and its plausibility. Early discussion with a radiologist will help to obtain the high-quality images required to investigate bony injury fully.

Case 6.6 Abdominal injury

Two-year-old Samson is attending the Emergency Department with his mother Kate. She says that he looked dreadful when she returned from work this evening and complained of tummy pain. Samson's step-father, who has looked after him today, told Kate that Samson had been fine all day.

On examination, Samson is very quiet and pale. He looks as if he is in severe pain and is lying very still on the bed. He avoids eye contact and flinches as you examine his abdomen. He is diffusely tender and there are some red marks and scratches on his abdomen. He is tachycardic.

Case 6.6 Exercise

◆ What would you do now?

◆ What are your concerns?

◆ Is this a typical presentation of physical abuse?

Case 6.6 Discussion

What would you do now?

Samson is shocked and needs resuscitating. You need to move him to the resuscitation area and get senior nursing and medical support. It may be appropriate to call the surgeons.

Samson needs close monitoring, oxygen, and intravenous access. You should take blood (including a cross-match) and commence intravenous fluids.

What are your concerns?

Samson is very unwell and immediate resuscitation is the priority. There are several worrying features. First, it is odd that Kate thought that he looked unwell as soon as she saw him, yet his step-father reported that he had been fine all day. Unlike accidental injury, where children are usually brought in immediately, in cases of inflicted injury it is common for children to present several hours after the event. Carers may report that the child was well and then suddenly became ill, which is unlikely in haemorrhagic shock or peritonitis.

Secondly, there are red marks and scratches on Samson's abdomen. These are not specific for non-accidental injury, but require explanation as it is unusual place for accidental injury. Blunt abdominal trauma can result in visible bruising, but this is not a consistent finding.

Is this a typical presentation of physical abuse?

Visceral injury is an uncommon form of physical child abuse. Signs and symptoms may mimic accidental injury and other abdominal pathology such as appendicitis. Often the diagnosis is not made until a child is operated on.

Most deliberate visceral injury is caused by blunt trauma and is most common in toddlers (Maguire et al., 2013). Though uncommon, it accounts for nearly half of deaths from physical abuse. It often occurs around the time of head injury in a child who has been badly beaten.

Case summary

Inflicted abdominal trauma is uncommon in children but carries a high mortality risk. It can present non-specifically and may look like appendicitis or other abdominal pathology. Active resuscitation is often needed, and senior medical and surgical colleagues must be involved early.

Conclusion

This chapter explores common forms of child physical abuse and demonstrates the central role of history and examination in detecting them. Physical abuse presents in a variety of ways, including poisoning and antenatal illicit drug use. It is important to stay vigilant for physical abuse in any encounter with children and young people to ensure that they are protected from further injury.

References

Bechtel, K., Stoessel, K., Leventhal, J.M., et al. (2004). Characteristics that distinguish accidental from abusive injury in hospitalized young children with head trauma. *Pediatrics*, **114**(1), 165–8.

Hinchcliffe, J. (2011). Forensic odontology, part 4. Human bite marks. *British Dental Journal*, **210**, 363–8.

Maguire, S.A., Mann, M. (2013). Systematic reviews of bruising in relation to child abuse—what have we learnt: an overview of review updates. *Evidence-Based Child Health*, **8**(2), 255–63.

Maguire, S.A., Moynihan, S., Mann, M., Potokar, T., Kemp, A.M. (2008). A systematic review of features which indicate intentional scalds in children. *Burns*, **34**(8), 1072–81.

Maguire, S.A., Upadhyaya, M., Evans, A., et al. (2013). A systematic review of abusive visceral injuries in childhood—their range and recognition. *Child Abuse and Neglect*, **37**(7), 430–45.

RCR/RCPCH (Royal College of Radiologists/Royal College of Paediatrics and Child Health). (2008). *Standards for Radiological Investigation of Suspected Non-accidental Injury*. London: Royal College of Paediatrics and Child Health.

7

Sexual abuse

Nirit Braha

Chapter summary

According to recent research, nearly a quarter of young adults have experienced some form of sexual abuse during their childhood, including contact and non-contact activities. Contact sexual abuse may include sexual touching as well as penetrative sex. Non-contact abuse may include sexual grooming, involving children in pornography, showing children images of sexual activity, and encouraging children to strip, masturbate, or engage in sexual activity with someone else. One in twenty children in the UK have experienced contact sexual abuse (Radford et al., 2011). Despite increased media and public awareness, sexual abuse remains largely a hidden problem and can be difficult to uncover. Many victims wait for years before telling anyone about their abuse as recently highlighted by Operation Yewtree and many other inquiries into institutional abuse.

Case 7.1 Acute sexual assault

Amy and Sarah are 14-year-old girls who have come to the Paediatric Emergency Department. Amy tells you that they were on their way home from school yesterday and met a 15-year-old friend, Tom, who offered them vodka. They went back to his house and the next thing Amy remembers is waking up on the sofa with no underwear and feeling sore. Sarah has brought Amy to the hospital because she is still sore and Sarah is worried about her. They haven't told their parents. Amy says that she has never had sex before. You offer to refer Amy to a Sexual Assault Referral Centre, but she declines. She also does not want you to call the police or tell her mother what has happened.

Case 7.1 Exercise

- Is this a crime?

- What do you need to do next?

- Should you ask Amy what happened?

- How would you examine Amy?

- What about forensic evidence?

- Should you call the police or speak to social care without Amy's consent?

- What else can you do for Amy?

Case 7.1 Discussion

Is this a crime?

Under the Sexual Offences Act 2003, if a child is under the age of 13 years, or is aged between 13 and 16 years and the perpetrator does not reasonably believe that the child is over 16 years, it is a criminal offence to:

- intentionally rape (the penetration by the penis of a child's vagina, anus, or mouth)

- sexually assault by penetration (penetrate sexually the vagina or anus of a child with a part of the body, such as a finger, or with anything else)

- sexually assault (touch sexually)

- cause or incite a child to engage in sexual activity.

For children under 13 years, whether or not the child consented to the act is irrelevant and is defined as statutory rape. The Crown Prosecution Service guidance (CPS, 2014) instructs that children between 13 and 16 years who are genuinely involved in consensual sexual relations should not be prosecuted.

Even though Tom is 15 years old, this was not a consensual act and should be reported to the police.

What do you need to do next?

You need to address Amy's health and psychosocial needs, and also consider the safeguarding and legal aspects of her case. Since Amy may have been raped, but has declined referral to a Sexual Assault Referral Centre, you can conduct a general paediatric assessment and offer her baseline screening for sexually transmitted infections and emergency contraception. Any injuries she has sustained should be assessed and treated. In addition, hepatitis B vaccination and post-exposure HIV prophylaxis should be considered. Although prophylaxis for chlamydia and gonorrhoea are not given routinely, it may be considered if Amy is felt to be unlikely to return for a follow-up appointment or is at high risk of infection (RCPCH, 2013). It is also important to explore Amy's social background, risk-taking behaviours, previous experiences of abuse, and need for counselling or other psychological support.

Should you ask Amy what happened?

If a child is going to give a statement to the police, it is preferable for this to happen before the medical assessment because anything they disclose during your assessment may form evidence in court, and inappropriate questioning can be seen as introducing new material or contaminating their evidence (RCPCH, 2008). This statement is taken by trained police officers, usually from the Child Abuse Investigation Team, and is referred to as an Achieving Best Evidence statement. When a child has already given a statement, there is no need to repeat taking the history of the assault.

As Amy has refused to speak to the police, you should ask open questions about what happened and for details relevant to your medical assessment.

How would you examine Amy?

After a thorough general examination, an anogenital examination should be undertaken with another professional acting as a chaperone (see Figure 7.1 for myths surrounding anogenital examination).

Three different positions can be used to examine Amy, as recommended in RCPCH (2008).

- Supine frog-leg position: the child lying on their back, with hips flexed and the soles of the feet touching.

- Prone knee–chest position: the child lying on their front, with their knees flexed and touching their chest. This should always follow examination in the frog-leg position in the prepubertal child if an abnormality is found in the posterior hymen.

◆ Lateral position: the child lying on their side, curled up with hips and knees flexed (for examining the anal region). Young children may be more comfortable held on a carer's lap with their back to the carer's chest.

You should look at the external genitalia and perianal region for erythema, bleeding, bruising, and any lacerations or abrasions. You should also look for discharge from the urethra, vagina, or anus, and for scar tissue or skin abnormalities. Then, you should gently separate the buttocks to assess the tone of the external sphincter and look for fissures, external haemorrhoids, skin tags, and warts. Both the internal and external anal sphincters may relax, with the anal canal opening up to reveal a clear view into the rectum. This is reflex anal dilatation and if noted should be interpreted carefully with reference to the latest evidence base.

The hymen should be inspected for lacerations, transections, and clefts—but these are best seen by a trained forensic physician using a colposcope. A colposcope is essentially a camera which allows still or video magnified images of the anus and genitalia. It is usually placed at the foot of the examination couch.

If you were examining a boy, you would look at the penis and scrotum. The foreskin would be gently retracted by you or the patient to view the urethral meatus and frenulum. The scrotum would be gently palpated to assess the presence of both testes and any pathology (RCPCH, 2008).

What about forensic evidence?

You can ask Amy for samples using an early evidence kit, which should be available in the Emergency Department or from the police. This kit contains a urine sample pot, a mouth swab, and mouth rinse. It allows early collection of DNA evidence and toxicology. When gathering samples, use chain of evidence (see Appendix 5 for an example template) so that any specimen presented as evidence in a court of law can be clearly demonstrated to have followed an unbroken chain from its source to the court. Each person who handles the sample, along with the places and conditions of storage, must be documented with the date, time, place, and signatures of custodians (BASHH, 2010). Most hospital laboratories have a designated chain of evidence staff member as well as a sealed refrigerator.

Should you call the police or speak to social care without Amy's consent?

You should explore Amy's reasons for declining referral to a Sexual Assault Referral Centre and asking you not to call the police. You should assess Amy's capacity to make this decision to refuse treatment (GMC, 2013). You should then discuss the case with the consultant paediatrician on call. If you decide that Amy is Gillick competent (NSPCC, 2014), you should respect her right

Myths surrounding paediatric Anogenital Examination

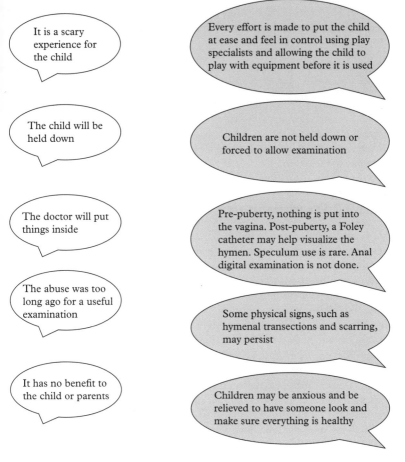

It is a scary experience for the child

Every effort is made to put the child at ease and feel in control using play specialists and allowing the child to play with equipment before it is used

The child will be held down

Children are not held down or forced to allow examination

The doctor will put things inside

Pre-puberty, nothing is put into the vagina. Post-puberty, a Foley catheter may help visualize the hymen. Speculum use is rare. Anal digital examination is not done.

The abuse was too long ago for a useful examination

Some physical signs, such as hymenal transections and scarring, may persist

It has no benefit to the child or parents

Children may be anxious and be relieved to have someone look and make sure everything is healthy

Figure 7.1 Myths surrounding the paediatric anogenital examination.

to confidentiality. Therefore you would not call the police unless you had good reason to believe that this would expose others to a risk of death or serious harm, for example from someone who is prepared to use weapons, or that others may be at risk (GMC, 2013). If Amy consents, you should refer to social care. If, from the history, you feel that she is still vulnerable, and at ongoing risk, you should breach confidentiality and refer to social care.

What else can you do for Amy?

You should strongly advise her to tell her parents what has happened. You should also offer her paediatric follow-up and a referral to the Child and Adolescent Mental Health Services.

Case summary

Acute cases of child sexual assault should be seen by a paediatrician or forensic physician who has the appropriate experience, equipment, and expertise to perform a forensic assessment. However, where Gillick competent children decline referral, it is still possible to ensure that their medical and psychosocial needs are met, and to obtain forensic evidence which could be used if they later report the crime to the police.

Case 7.2 Straddle injury

Anna, aged seven, presents to the Emergency Department with bleeding and vulval pain in the late evening. She is very tearful and distressed. Her mother says that Anna jumped from one bed to another in her bedroom, and fell awkwardly onto the wooden bed frame. Anna is crying and refusing to let anyone approach her. Her pyjama bottoms are blood-stained. A nurse gently coaxes Anna into allowing her to perform some basic observations, which establish that Anna is haemodynamically stable. She gives Anna some pain relief, which soothes her and helps a little with the pain.

Meanwhile, you take a history from Anna's mother who confirms that she was in the room at the time of the incident and brought Anna to the hospital immediately. Despite analgesia, reassurance, and support from her mother, Anna is very distressed and unable to tolerate any more than a cursory inspection. You are unable to see the origin of the bleeding but there is only a small amount of blood on the swab she is holding. She has passed urine and there is 1+ of blood on dipstick testing.

> ## Case 7.2 Exercise
>
> ◆ What are your priorities?
>
> ◆ Does she need an examination under anaesthesia?
>
> ◆ How should you manage her injury?

Case 7.2 Discussion

What are your priorities?

You need to stop Anna's bleeding and treat her pain, and, if possible, determine the nature and extent of her injuries and whether she needs surgery. Here, the history is consistent with the presentation, and you have no safeguarding concerns.

Does Anna need an examination under anaesthesia?

When a Gillick competent child refuses examination, it should not be done. Options include further explanation and reassurance, or scheduling a follow-up appointment to allow time for a rapport to build up between the paediatrician and the child. If a child does not have sufficient understanding *and* it is in their best interests, then examination may proceed with parental consent, but the justification for this must be clearly documented in the medical records (RCPCH, 2008).

In this situation, where the child is young and too frightened to understand what is happening and give consent, you still would not hold Anna down to force examination but would consider whether an examination under anaesthesia was necessary instead. This should be considered where children are unable to tolerate examination, there is suspicion of an injury not visualized by an external examination, or there is clinical suspicion of sexual abuse and a more detailed examination is needed (RCPCH, 2008). In this case, Anna is stable and there is no evidence of severe haemorrhage or significant ongoing bleeding.

You feel that she is likely to cooperate with an examination by a specialist in the morning, under calmer, more child-centred conditions. The case is discussed with the consultant on call and with social care. The consultant agrees that an examination under anaesthesia is not currently required, but advises that it would be necessary if Anna were to experience more severe bleeding. Anna is admitted to the ward for observation overnight. The duty social worker confirms that Anna is not known to social care.

How should you manage her injury?

Where bleeding is mild or has stopped, and the child can pass urine and faeces spontaneously, management of straddle injuries includes simple analgesia, irrigation with warm water, and compression with gauze swabs. Following discharge, salt-water baths and ice packs can be used, together with topical anaesthetic cream or barrier creams to reduce pain on micturition. In more severe cases, where there is ongoing bleeding, the child is unable to void, or the history is not consistent with the injuries seen, the child should be discussed with a paediatric gynaecologist or urologist and may need surgical treatment and a urethral catheter (Royal Children's Hospital Melbourne, 2014).

Case summary

Straddle injuries are common but should always provoke consideration of whether the history fits the presentation seen. Children should not be held down for anogenital examination. In cases of severe bleeding, or where there is suspicion of a deeper injury or of sexual abuse, an examination under anaesthesia may become necessary. In milder cases, children may respond better to examination under calmer conditions in the daytime once their pain and distress have settled.

Case 7.3 Sexualized behaviour

Arik, a ten-year-old boy, is referred to paediatric outpatients by his GP. His teachers have expressed concerns about his behaviour in class over the last six months. He has been found in the playground showing his penis to classmates and forcing younger girls to imitate sexual acts despite repeatedly being asked to stop. Arik becomes angry when he is asked to focus on the lesson or told that it is not acceptable to masturbate in public. These behaviours have caused the other children in his class to avoid him. His mother is also concerned because he has appeared withdrawn and secretive at home and has started wetting the bed.

Case 7.3 Exercise

◆ How likely is Arik's behaviour to be secondary to sexual abuse?

◆ Are there any other worrying features in the history?

◆ Is there anything else you would like to know?

◆ What should happen next?

Case 7.3 Discussion

How likely is Arik's behaviour to be secondary to sexual abuse?

Sexual behaviours are common in children. Sexual behaviours in children between two and five years include touching their genitals at home and in public, showing their genitals to others, and trying to look at nude peers and adults. These behaviours are generally transient and distractible. The variety and frequency of sexual behaviours increases up to five years of age and decreases thereafter. Older children with developmental disorders may exhibit these sexual behaviours because they do not understand that it is socially inappropriate (Kellogg, 2009).

Sexual behaviour problems are behaviours that are 'developmentally inappropriate, intrusive or abusive' (Kellogg, 2009). Sexual abuse, physical abuse, and neglect are a common but not exclusive experience among children with sexual behaviour problems. There are several 'red flag' signs to look for in the history. These include persistent or coercive behaviours, a large age gap between the children involved, and explicit imitation of sexual acts. Behaviours such as inserting objects into genitalia and touching the genitalia of animals are also uncommon and may be cause for concern. Parents' reactions can escalate sexual behaviours. Therefore parents are advised not to punish or admonish the child for normative sexual behaviours, but instead to use gentle distraction (Kellogg, 2009). Where behaviours are not settling despite parental redirection, further assessment by a mental health professional should be considered, together with referral to social care if abuse or neglect is suspected.

Are there any other worrying features in the history?

Arik is bedwetting again and has appeared secretive and withdrawn. These are also features of emotional distress in children and merit further assessment.

Is there anything else you would like to know?

As well as a detailed history, you will need to ask about Arik's development and any previous behavioural concerns. You should also take a detailed family history, including any recent changes or stressors, and ask whether Arik has access to pornographic material or witnesses sexual activities at home or elsewhere (Kellogg, 2009).

What should happen next?

You elicit a history of sexual behaviour that is coercive and causes emotional distress to others, together with other behavioural changes suggestive of distress. Therefore Arik requires a safeguarding assessment. His case should be discussed with the consultant paediatrician on call and a referral made to children's social care.

Case summary

Sexual behaviours are common in children and are part of normal development. However, persistent or coercive behaviours, large differences in age between children, and explicit imitation of sexual acts can be markers of sexual abuse and may warrant further investigation.

Case 7.4 Vaginal discharge

A nine-year-old girl, Aisha, is referred to paediatric outpatients with a six-month history of a thin white vaginal discharge, itchiness, and soreness. Vulval swabs from her GP have been negative. A course of clotrimazole cream has made no difference to her symptoms. Aisha is otherwise a well child, who is described as happy and doing well at school. There are no concerns about her mood or behaviour. You examine Aisha and see a small amount of white discharge, erythema around the vaginal introitus, and some excoriation marks.

Case 7.4 Exercise

- When is vaginal discharge normal?

- What is the differential diagnosis?

- How would you treat Aisha?

- What if the discharge is purulent or persists despite treatment?

Case 7.4 Discussion

When is vaginal discharge normal?

Newborn girls may have a thick mucous discharge, which can be blood-stained, due to maternal oestrogen stimulation of the vaginal mucosa, cervical epithelium, and endometrium. This disappears within 7–10 days. Between six months and a year prior to menarche, the increase in oestrogen levels causes a grey–white discharge, which is not irritating and not offensive (Sharma et al., 2004). Once girls have started their periods, they may have a clear or white discharge, which varies with their menstrual cycle, and may also have a slightly brownish discharge at the end of their periods.

What is the differential diagnosis?

These symptoms are typical of a non-specific vulvovaginitis. It is the most common gynaecological problem affecting pre-pubertal girls. The hypo-oestrogenic hormonal milieu predisposes the vaginal mucosa to infection and inflammation. Symptoms include vaginal discharge, vulval soreness, pruritus, bleeding, and dysuria (Joishy et al., 2005).

Other causes of vaginal pruritus or discharge include beta-haemolytic *Streptococcus* or *Haemophilus influenzae* infection, *Enterobius vermicularis* (threadworms), lichen sclerosus, and labial adhesions. Vaginal discharge may also result from sexually transmitted infections or a vaginal foreign body. Candidal vulvovaginitis is very uncommon in prepubertal children who no longer wear nappies. Physical signs of vulvovaginitis include inflammation with erythema of the introitus; excoriation of the genital area, and vaginal discharge (Joishy et al., 2005).

How would you treat Aisha?

After a detailed history and examination, swabs of vaginal secretions from the introitus can be sent for culture and antibiotics offered only if a pathogen is identified. For non-specific vulvovaginitis, helpful measures include advising girls to wipe front to back after using the toilet and avoidance of bubble baths, perfumes, and biological detergents. Parents should be told that douching (cleaning inside the vagina) is unnecessary and counterproductive, as the vagina is self-cleaning. Children should be advised to wear loose cotton underwear, and avoid wearing tights, tight trousers, and underwear at night (Joishy et al., 2005). Salt-water baths and bland emollients such as E45, Sudocrem, and zinc cream can be used to soothe the area during flare-ups.

What if the discharge is purulent or persistent despite treatment?

This should prompt consideration of a sexually transmitted infection, a vaginal foreign body, or a resistant organism. Perineal pruritus which is worse at night should prompt consideration of *Enterobius* infection.

Case summary

Vaginal discharge is a frequent presentation. Even though non-specific vulvovaginitis is the most common cause, the differential diagnosis includes vaginal foreign bodies or a sexually transmitted infection resulting from sexual abuse. A careful history should be taken, looking for concerning features such as purulent or persistent discharge, aggressive, hostile, or withdrawn behaviour, frequent absences from school, or sexual behaviour problems. In most cases, non-specific vulvovaginitis will respond well to hygiene measures and reassurance.

Case 7.5 Historical sexual abuse

Aidan, seven years old, discloses to his mother, Sue, that their lodger, James, has penetrated him anally with his finger and his penis when his mother was at work. James moved out three months ago. Aidan didn't tell his mother before because James threatened that he would hurt her if he told anyone. Aidan's mother, shocked and unsure what to do, takes him to their GP and asks for advice.

Case 7.5 Exercise

◆ What should the GP do next?

◆ Should the GP question Aidan about what happened?

◆ Should the GP examine Aidan?

◆ What else can the GP do for Aidan and his family?

Case 7.5 Discussion

What should the GP do next?

Aidan has disclosed historic sexual abuse. The GP should follow local protocols, including making a referral to social care who will arrange for an early assessment at a local safeguarding clinic. There, Aidan would undergo a full paediatric assessment including anogenital examination and screening for sexually transmitted infections. This is statutory rape, and the police should also be informed. In general, the Child Abuse Investigation Team would be called by social care and an investigation begun into the criminal aspects of this case.

Should the GP question Aidan about what happened?

The Child Abuse Investigation Team will probably arrange for Aidan to have an Achieving Best Evidence interview. To avoid any suggestion of contaminating Aidan's evidence, the GP should only ask open questions as needed to establish whether Aidan has any symptoms requiring medical attention.

Should the GP examine Aidan?

Aidan should be examined by a paediatrician or forensic physician with appropriate knowledge, skills, and experience (RCPCH, 2013). There is no need for the GP to examine him as well, unless he has symptoms that need urgent attention. Aidan is at risk of sexually transmitted infections and these should be addressed as in Case 7.1.

What else can the GP do for Aidan and his family?

The GP could offer Aidan and his mother referral for psychological support.

Case summary

In cases of historic sexual abuse, when over 72 hours have elapsed since the last episode and the child is not in need of immediate medical intervention, a referral should be made to social care who will coordinate an early paediatric forensic assessment and inform the police. This means that a child receives care and attention from those professionals best equipped to meet the child's health and social needs as well as gathering forensic evidence for a prosecution.

Conclusion

Putting the pieces of the puzzle together to correctly diagnose child sexual abuse is a challenging multidisciplinary endeavour. Victims may not disclose their abuse for many years, as highlighted by recent high-profile prosecutions of celebrities. This chapter describes an approach to the sexually abused child, as well as common presentations where child sexual abuse is among the differential diagnoses. Whether or not a disclosure of sexual abuse has been made, thorough yet sensitive history-taking and examination by an experienced professional can do much to protect the child from further harm.

Please note at the time of going to press the RCPCH (2008) guidance on the Physical Signs of Sexual Abuse was being updated but not yet published. The authors would advise readers who perform sexual abuse examinations to ensure they are familiar with the changes and evidence base in this update.

References

BASSH (Clinical Effectiveness Group, British Association for Sexual Health and HIV). (2010). *United Kingdom Guideline on the Management of Sexually Transmitted Infections and Related Conditions in Children and Young People—2010*. Available at: http://www.bashh.org/documents/2674.pdf (accessed 14 July 2014).

CPS (Crown Prosecution Service). (2014). *Rape and Sexual Offences: Legal Guidance*. Available at: http://www.cps.gov.uk/legal/p_to_r/rape_and_sexual_offences/ (accessed 14 July 2014).

GMC (General Medical Council). (2013). *Good Medical Practice (2013)*. Available at: http://www.gmc-uk.org/guidance/good_medical_practice.asp (accessed 14 July 2014).

Sexual Offences Act 2003 (c.42). London: HMSO.

Gray D., Watt P. (2013). *Giving Victims a Voice: Joint report into the sexual allegations against Jimmy Savile*. London: NSPCC. Available at: http://www.nspcc.org.uk/globalassets/documents/research-reports/yewtree-report-giving-victims-voice-jimmy-savile.pdf (accessed 03 November 2015).

Joishy M., Ashtekar, C.S., Jain, A., Gonsalves, R. (2005). Do we need to treat vulvovaginitis in prepubertal girls? *British Medical Journal*, **330**(7484), 186–8.

Kellogg, N.D. (2009). Clinical Report: The evaluation of sexual behaviours in children. *Pediatrics*, **124**, 992–8.

NSPCC (National Society for the Prevention of Cruelty to Children) (2014). *Gillick Competency and Fraser Guidelines. NSPCC Factsheet*. Available at: http://www.nspcc.org.uk/inform/research/questions/gillick_wda61289.html (accessed 28 September 2014).

Radford, L., Corral, S., Bradley, C., et al. (2011). *Child Abuse and Neglect in the UK Today*. London: NSPCC. Available at: http://www.nspcc.org.uk/Inform/research/findings/child_abuse_neglect_research_PDF_wdf84181.pdf (accessed 14 July 2014).

Royal Children's Hospital Melbourne. (2014) *Clinical Practice Guidelines: Straddle Injuries*. Available at: http://www.rch.org.au/clinicalguide/guideline_index/Straddle_Injuries/ (accessed on 14/07/2014).

RCPCH (Royal College of Paediatrics and Child Health). (2008). *The Physical Signs of Child Sexual Abuse: An Evidence-Based Review and Guidance for Best Practice*. Lavenham, Suffolk: Lavenham Press. Available at: http://www.rcpch.ac.uk/physical-signs-child-sexual-abuse (accessed 28 September 2014).

RCPCH (Royal College of Paediatrics and Child Health). (2013). *Child Protection Companion* (2nd edn). Available at: http://www.rcpch.ac.uk/child-protection-companion (accessed 14 July 2014).

Sexual Offences Act 2003 (c.42). London: HMSO.

Sharma, B., Preston, J., Greenwood, P. (2004). Management of vulvovaginitis and vaginal discharge in prepubertal girls. *Reviews in Gynaecological Practice*, 4, 111–20.

Finding your nearest Sexual Assault Referral Centre

NHS Choices website: https://www.nhs.uk/Service-Search/Rape-and-sexual-assault-referral-centres/LocationSearch/364

8

Emotional abuse

Charlotte Holland

Chapter summary

Emotional abuse is common, and can occur alone or in conjunction with other forms of abuse. It occurs when there is persistent psychological maltreatment, leading to an adverse effect on the child. Abuse can happen in many environments, but frequently within the home. It can be active, for example rejection or exploitation, or passive, including emotional unavailability or negative interactions. Signs of emotional abuse can be subtle and age-dependent. Children may present with physical manifestations of stress, such as secondary enuresis or self-harm, or strange behaviours including aggression or submissiveness. They may be referred because of developmental delay or anxiety. Recognition and management of emotional abuse is vital to prevent long-term sequelae.

Emotional abuse: definition and patterns

Emotional abuse, also termed psychological maltreatment, was the reason for a 'child protection' or 'child in need' plan in 28 per cent of cases for England and Wales in 2012 (NSPCC, 2013). There is an emotional component to all forms of abuse, but emotional abuse can occur in isolation. It is difficult to quantify, particularly as the main cause of abuse, and can be hard to identify.

Emotional abuse is defined as 'persistent emotional maltreatment of children such as to cause severe and persistent adverse effects on the child's emotional development. It may involve conveying to children that they are worthless or unloved, inadequate or valued only insofar as they meet the needs of another person' (HM Government, 2006).

Patterns of emotional abuse (see Table 8.1) may be active or passive (Barlow and Scrader-MacMillan, 2009; Glaser, 2011; Hibbard et al., 2012). Active emotional abuse implies a premeditated intention to cause harm, including trying to scare, demean, or verbally abuse, sarcasm, or singling a child out for punishment or humiliation. It may involve refusing to acknowledge the child or

Table 8.1 Patterns of emotional abuse

Active (acts of commission)	Passive (acts of omission)
Spurning/rejecting	Emotional unavailability or ignoring child
Terrorizing	Negative attitudes
Isolating	Developmentally inappropriate interaction with child
Exploiting or corrupting	Failure to recognize child's individuality
	Failure to promote social adaption

show affection, or isolation by denying the child normal social experiences (e.g. locking in a bedroom). Other examples of active emotional abuse include corruption of the child by creating a destructive or antisocial environment, sexual exploitation, or reinforcing deviant behaviour.

Passive abuse involves denying love and care. This includes ignoring the child, denying access to essential activities for stimulation and interaction, or lack of protection from danger. It may be secondary to negative influences within the home, for example domestic violence. It also encompasses developmentally inappropriate interactions with the child, for example continual criticism or overly advanced expectations of the child's behaviour and accomplishments.

Case 8.1 Recurrent abdominal pain

You are asked to see Susan, 12 years old, who presents to the Emergency Department for the third time with abdominal pain. She has severe central pain with radiation to the back and epigastrium which has lasted for three weeks. On examination, findings were inconsistent, with reported pain and voluntary guarding out of proportion with clinical observation. Her GP prescribed omeprazole two weeks ago which has not resolved symptoms.

You admit her to the paediatric ward for observation. Her pain does not settle with simple analgesics. Urine dipstick, abdominal X-ray, and ultrasound are normal. You talk to Susan to clarify history and explain endoscopy, and she confides that she is having difficulties at home. She disclosed that her parents shout and physically fight with each other. Her mother frequently comments on Susan's weight and appearance, and demands unachievable goals for school work. It appears that her mother demonstrates symptoms suggestive of obsessive–compulsive disorder with excessive cleanliness. Susan's mother expects her to help with cooking and housework every evening. She also divulges she is being bullied at school.

Case 8.1 Exercise

♦ What clinical points are suggestive of emotional abuse in this case?

♦ How can emotional abuse present?

♦ Does emotional abuse only occur in the home?

♦ What are the consequences of emotional abuse?

♦ What should you do next for Susan?

♦ Can emotional abuse be resolved?

Case 8.1 Discussion

What clinical points are suggestive of emotional abuse in this case?

Susan has many stressors in her life. She has sought medical advice on multiple occasions for real symptoms of pain, but the cause of the pain is probably psychological. She has low self-esteem, compounded by the attitudes of her mother and bullying at school. Other household risk factors include parental mental health issues and domestic violence.

How can emotional abuse present?

Signs of emotional abuse can be subtle and age-dependent. General health and well-being should be examined; a decline in growth velocity can be an indicator of ill-treatment or neglect. Delay in reaching developmentally appropriate milestones can be indicators of lack of environmental stimulation or attention (Glaser, 2011; NSPCC, 2013; RCPCH, 2013). Presentation may be in the Emergency Department, in the outpatient setting, in primary care, or at school.

The first signs of suspicion may be observation of negative interactions between parent and child, with lack of attachment to the caregiver. As the consultation progresses, they may demonstrate abnormal behaviours or physical manifestations of stress. This may only emerge after a further in-depth history following referral for a medical concern. Difficult behaviours are often used as a coping strategy for dealing with emotional abuse, and are not the child 'being naughty'. Glaser (2011) suggests the following presentations:

♦ Behavioural manifestations:

○ abnormally passive or lethargic

○ indiscriminate attention-seeking

- ○ aggression or oppositional behaviour
- ○ faecal smearing
- ○ absconding from home or school
- ○ antisocial behaviours, low empathy
- ○ substance misuse.

♦ Physical manifestations:
- ○ sleep disturbance
- ○ excessive drinking or pica
- ○ soiling or secondary enuresis
- ○ gratification through food
- ○ self-mutilation
- ○ non-organic pain.

♦ Possible referrals
- ○ developmental delay
- ○ disproportionate weight and height with no medical explanation
- ○ eating disorders
- ○ school failure
- ○ anxiety or depression
- ○ psychosomatic disease.

It is important to consider emotional abuse in any of these presentations or if anything strikes you as 'not quite right' with the child's behaviour, history given, or caregiver–child interactions. A comprehensive social history will help identify risk factors for emotional abuse (Dong et al., 2004).

Does emotional abuse only occur in the home?

Emotional abuse usually involves the primary caregivers, however can occur in other settings. Cultural values may play a part. Examples of emotionally abusive environments include the following:

♦ **Home**: domestic violence, attachment disorders, inappropriate parental responses, fabricated or induced illness.

♦ **School**: bullying, cyberbullying, prevention of attendance.

♦ **Other**: exploitation of children as sex workers, trafficking, forced marriage.

What are the consequences of emotional abuse?

Emotional abuse, either alone or in conjunction with other forms of abuse, can cause wide-reaching and long-term consequences for the child, affecting attachment, education, and social and behavioural areas of development. It may depend on the exact nature and length of abuse, but the effect on the child cannot be predicted (Glaser, 2011). Psychological maltreatment in the first three years of life may be of particular concern, as there is rapid brain growth and developmental milestones to achieve which may be adversely affected by the environment (Hibbard et al., 2012).

In the short term, the child may suffer from a range of physical and psychological difficulties, including growth failure, low self-esteem, anxiety, and depression.

Long-term consequences involve poor adaptation to adult life and relationships. Studies have shown that multiple adverse childhood experiences, for example child abuse, neglect, or witnessing domestic violence, are associated with many health problems later in life, including smoking, substance misuse, liver disease, poor marital or parenting skills, unintended pregnancies, sexually transmitted diseases, suicide attempts, and other psychiatric illness (Barlow and Scrader-MacMillan, 2009; Wolfe and McIsaac, 2011).

What should you do next for Susan?

It can be difficult to recognize or pinpoint possible emotional abuse. It may be possible from a single admission, or require repeated observations of family dynamics and interactions in different settings (RCPCH, 2013) (see Box 8.1). The aims are to stop maltreatment, prevent recurrence, and manage or negate harmful effects (Glaser, 2011).

Discussion with Susan's parents should be non-accusatory and non-judgemental, with her health and emotional well-being as the central focus. Her parents may not be aware of the consequences of their behaviours or attitudes. A full social history should be taken. It can be difficult to collate tangible evidence. If chronic emotional abuse is suspected but immediate removal from the environment is not thought to be in the child's best interests, referral to social care is still

---

Box 8.1 Initial actions in suspected emotional abuse

- History from child alone as well as with caregiver
- Discussion with senior
- Are they known to social care? Discuss with duty social worker
- Does the child need immediate removal to a place of safety?
- Involvement of local child protection team

required. Social workers, health visitors, and clinical psychologists can provide ongoing assessment, with observation of the child and family interactions in different environments.

Can emotional abuse be resolved?

Prevention of further abuse is paramount. Various specific interventions are described, but evaluation of and the evidence base for interventions are poor (Barlow and Scrader-MacMillan, 2009; Glaser, 2011). Programmes including several sessions with a clear behavioural focus may be most effective. Intervention styles include the following (Hibbard et al., 2012):

◆ **Parent-focused**: aimed at changing an aspect of parent's well-being or parenting style that is contributing to emotionally abusive interactions, including cognitive behavioural programmes, short-term crisis or longer-term interventions, home visits, or full residential programmes.

◆ **Parent- and child-focused**: directed at changing parent–child interactions, including psychotherapeutic approaches, or video guidance with discussion and education.

◆ **Family-focused**: aimed at changing aspects of family functioning, including input from social care or child and adolescent mental health services.

The type of intervention required can be adapted according to the pattern of emotional abuse. Glaser (2011) describes five categories of abuse and suggests therapeutic interventions for which there is some evidence (see Table 8.2).

Prevention of emotional abuse before it occurs would be the ultimate achievement. Population-based approaches, for example the UK Healthy Child Programme, recommend that all contact between professionals and parents should be used as an opportunity to promote parenting skills and attachment, and to identify concerns or risk factors that may need further input (Barlow and Scrader-MacMillan, 2009). Targeted approaches include identification of at-risk groups and use of a range of interventions to improve home environment, access to services, and development of child–caregiver interactions, for example in Sure Start centres. The most appropriate intervention may depend on the individual family, but will often require a multidisciplinary approach (Hibbard et al., 2012; Wolfe and McIsaac, 2011).

Conclusion

Emotional abuse is common, either alone or in conjunction with other forms of abuse. It involves repeated patterns of damaging interactions between child and caregiver, and can take many forms. Emotional abuse should be considered

Table 8.2 Interventions in emotional abuse

Category	Root of abuse	Interventions used
Emotional unavailability	Caregiver often has own difficulties which stop them from responding appropriately to the child	◆ Identify and manage risk factors (e.g. substance misuse, mental health disorders, domestic violence) ◆ Parent- and child-focused work: encouraging good attachment and interactions
Negative attributions	Caregiver has negative beliefs about child (e.g. their temperament or personality)	◆ Parent-focused work: build up rapport and explore views or personal difficulties to arrive at solutions
Inappropriate developmental expectations, domestic violence, and inconsistent and /or harsh parenting	Caregiver unaware of child's developmental needs, or how to set boundaries or provide consistent care	◆ Psycho-educational parenting approach and training
Using child for fulfilment of caregiver's needs (includes fabricating illness)	Caregiver unable to distinguish psychological boundary between the child and themselves	◆ Identify contributing factors (e.g. unresolved partner conflict, serious maltreatment in caregiver's past or present) ◆ Parent-focused work to change these factors and understand implications for the child
Failure to promote socialization	Caregiver unaware of the effect of lack of interactions with peers, environment, and themselves	◆ Multidisciplinary team approach ◆ Parent and child or family focused

in children with new behaviour changes, school failure, or unexplained failure to thrive. Prevention of emotional abuse by population-based and targeted interventions such as parenting groups at Sure Start centres may be beneficial. Emotional abuse can take a long time to identify, but when it is identified, an individualized approach is required. Interventions for which there is evidence of effectiveness include cognitive behavioural parenting programmes or other psychotherapeutic interventions.

References

Barlow, J., Scrader-MacMillan, A. (2009). *Safeguarding Children from Emotional Abuse—What Works? Research Brief*. Available at: https://www.gov.uk/government/uploads/system/uploads/attachment_data/file/222093/DCSF-RBX-09-09.pdf (accessed 5 October 2014).

Dong, M., Anda, R.F., Felitte, V.J., et al. (2004). The interrelatedness of multiple forms of childhood abuse, neglect, and household dysfunction. *Child Abuse & Neglect*, **28**(7), 771–84.

Glaser, D. (2011). How to deal with emotional abuse and neglect—further development of a conceptual framework (FRAMEA). *Child Abuse & Neglect*, **35** (10), 866–75.

HM Government. (2006). Working Together to Safeguard Children. London: TSO

Hibbard, R., Barlow, J., Macmillan, H., et al. (2012). Psychological maltreatment. *Pediatrics*, **130**(2), 372–8.

NSPCC (National Society for the Prevention of Cruelty to Children). (2013). *Emotional Abuse: NSPCC Research Briefing*. Available at: http://www.nspcc.org.uk/Inform/research/briefings/emotionalabuse_wda48215.html (accessed 28 November 2013).

RCPCH (Royal College of Paediatrics and Child Health). (2013). *Child Protection Companion* (2nd edn). Lavenham, Suffolk: Lavenham Press.

Wolfe, D.A., McIsaac, C. (2011). Distinguishing between poor/dysfunctional parenting and child emotional maltreatment. *Child Abuse & Neglect*, **35**(10), 802–13.

9

Neglect

Eleanor Beagley and Gayle Hann

Chapter summary

Neglect is the most common type of abuse, as well as one of the most difficult to recognize. Signs are often subtle, and no exact threshold has been set for when a parent's level of care is unacceptable. This chapter will cover the extent and types of neglect, as well as how to identify it, by highlighting concerning features within cases.

Introduction: the extent of the problem

Neglect is the most common form of abuse, totalling 41 per cent of child protection registrations in the UK. On 31 March 2012 21,666 children in the UK were on child protection plans under a category that included neglect (Department for Education, 2013). It is estimated that one in seven secondary school children have been neglected at some point, with one in ten severely neglected (Radford et al., 2011). Despite being the most common form of abuse, neglect is also one of the hardest to recognize. Signs are often subtle, and no exact threshold has been set for when a parent's level of care is unacceptable. Therefore it is up to the individual health professional to make their own interpretation of the case and ascertain whether intervention is needed. Failure to respond to a child's basic needs can affect all areas of development, so it is crucial that risk factors are not ignored (see Table 9.1).

Types of neglect

Neglect can be subdivided into categories:

♦ **Medical neglect:** parent or carer fails to meet the medical needs of the child, either by not seeking medical attention when appropriate or failing to administer necessary medications.

♦ **Emotional neglect:** long-term emotional unavailability from a parent or carer towards the child.

Table 9.1 Concerning features suggesting neglect.

Physical features	Emotional and behavioural features
Severe and persistent infestations (scabies, head lice)	Child is withdrawn, fearful, or has low self-esteem
Consistently inappropriate clothing or footwear	Child is aggressive or oppositional
Poor hygiene (persistently smelly and dirty)	Indiscriminate contact or affection seeking
Untreated health problems (dental caries) or failure to engage with child health promotion programmes (immunizations)	Late attainment of developmental milestones
Faltering growth due to lack of provision of an adequate or appropriate diet	Self-stimulating (such as rocking) or self-injurious behaviour
Injury (burn or ingestion of harmful substance) that suggests lack of appropriate supervision	Child has regular responsibilities that interfere with essential normal daily activities (school)

Adapted from NICE, (2009).

◆ **Nutritional neglect:** provision of inadequate food or nutrition to support normal growth, as well as providing consistently unhealthy meals which can lead to obesity (see Chapter 10, Case 10.4).

◆ **Physical neglect:** inappropriate or unsafe living arrangements, dirty bedding or clothes, and poor personal hygiene.

◆ **Educational neglect:** parents or carers fail to enrol their child in school, discourage attendance, or fail to take an interest in education or support their child's learning needs.

◆ **Supervision:** parent or carer fails to provide adequate supervision to keep the child safe.

Case 9.1 Failure to thrive

You are a GP seeing a six-week-old boy for his routine baby check. Kian was born at term via normal vaginal delivery weighing 3.5 kg (25th centile). He was discharged on day one after a normal baby check. When you weigh Kian today, he is 3.64 kg (2nd centile). You note in the Personal Child Health Record ('red book') that when he was four days old he was visited by the midwife and weighed 3.40 kg (see Figure 9.1). His mother, Victoria, reports that he is exclusively breastfed and that he cries all the time and she is getting very little sleep. The health visitor visited when he was ten days old and had no concerns. You examine Kian and, apart from some mild nappy rash, he seems well. You ask Victoria if she has help from her partner, but she says that they broke up before Kian was born because of domestic violence. Victoria seems low in mood, but denies this and says that she is just tired.

Case 9.1 Exercise

- What are your concerns?

- Are there any concerning features for neglect in the history?

- Are there any concerning signs of neglect in the examination?

- What should you do next?

Case 9.1 Discussion:

What are your concerns?

Although it can be normal for growth to fluctuate, particularly during their first year of life, crossing centiles is still a concern. Failure to thrive describes a child who is not achieving the expected rate of growth for their age. Poor weight gain in a baby has many causes, and so it is important to first rule out any organic cause of Kian's decreased rate of growth.

Are there any concerning features for neglect in the history?

- Kian's history has no suggestion of any underlying illness, which should raise the question of an inorganic cause or possibly neglect.

- Although Victoria denies having a low mood, she may be finding her lack of sleep difficult to cope with. It is possible that this has evoked a negative response and she has become less emotionally attuned to Kian's needs, manifesting in him being malnourished.

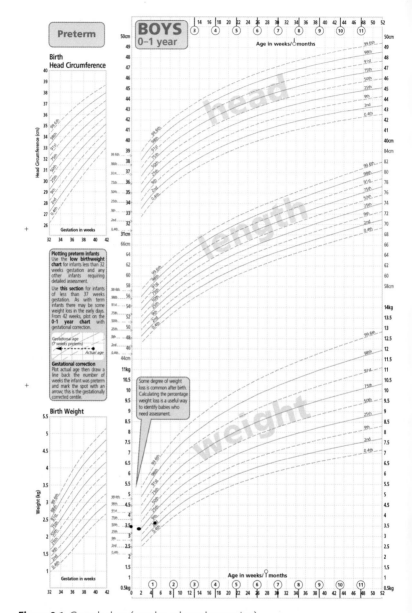

Figure 9.1 Growth chart (see also colour plate section).

Reproduced with permission from Royal College of Paediatric and Child Health, *Early years - UK-WHO growth charts and resources, Preterm Boys 0-1 year*, UK-WHO Chart 2009, Copyright © DH Copyright 2009, available from http://www.rcpch.ac.uk/system/files/protected/page/A4%20 Boys%200-4YRS%20(4th%20Jan%202013).pdf

- Victoria is a single mother. We don't know how old she is, but if she is also young these risk factors may combine to make neglect more likely.

- Domestic violence is also a parental risk factor for neglect. Although Victoria is no longer with her partner, it is still something to take into account when thinking about the family's history and the impact this might have had.

Are there any concerning signs of neglect in the examination?

On examination, Kian seems well with only mild nappy rash found. In isolation this would not suggest neglect, but because of Kian's history it is important to keep it in mind.

What should you do next?

- Victoria should be assessed for postnatal depression.

- Kian is exclusively breastfed. Victoria could be advised to express to determine what her milk supply is like and also top up with formula until the next review. If Kian gains weight with formula top-ups, an organic cause for failure to thrive is unlikely.

- You do not have any solid evidence of neglect at this stage, but could ask the health visitor to perform a home visit to re-weigh Kian and assess the home environment.

Case summary

Every opportunity should be taken to record a child's growth in their Personal Child Health Record ('red book') to ensure that any abnormalities are detected before the child's health and development are permanently affected. If poor growth is found and an organic cause is ruled out, neglect should always be considered.

Case 9.2 Physical neglect

It is midday in the Emergency Department (ED). You have been asked to see eight-year-old Ben, who has presented with a superficial burn to his right hand. When you ask him how it happened, he says he accidentally touched the hob in the kitchen when preparing breakfast. Ben is with his 14-year-old sister, Susie. You ask where their parents are and Susie tells you that they have been alone in the house since the previous afternoon, and that she doesn't know where they have gone. You find out later that Ben has already been seen in the Emergency Department three times in the last two months.

Case 9.2 Exercise

- Are there any concerning features in the history?

- What should you do next?

- Are these children being neglected?

Case 9.2 Discussion

Are there any concerning features in the history?

- An eight-year-old has been left in the care of a 14-year-old for nearly 24 hours. It is worrying enough in isolation, but if this is a regular occurrence, then it is concerning for neglect (see Chapter 2 for the law on leaving children in charge of younger children).

- Ben's injury is concerning and suggests a lack of appropriate supervision.

- Ben has been seen unusually frequently in the Emergency Department recently. This may have a simple explanation, but until you know why, this is also a cause for concern.

- It is midday, and neither Ben nor Susie are at school. Regularly missing or not being able to go to school may be a feature of neglect.

See Table 9.1 for more concerning features of neglect.

What should you do next?

- The parents should be contacted to find out why they were absent for nearly 24 hours. Ideally they should come to the hospital so that a full family and social history can be obtained.

- You should check to see if Ben and Susie are on a child protection plan.

- You should find out the reasons for Ben's previous attendances.

- You should contact the school to find out what the children's attendance record is like and whether the school has concerns.

You discover that Susie and Ben's parents are both struggling with mental health problems. Both children have poor school attendance, and teachers report that

Susie often becomes very aggressive and oppositional with minor provocation. Questions were raised last time Ben was seen in the Emergency Department, but the children are not currently subject to a child protection plan.

Are these children being neglected?

◆ There is no minimum age in the UK at which a child can be left on their own (see Chapter 2). However, it is possible to prosecute parents for neglect if in leaving a child they are putting them at risk of danger to their health (Children and Young Persons Act, 1933). In Ben's case it is clear that his health has been put at significant risk due to lack of appropriate supervision.

◆ Parental mental health issues should not lead you to assume that they are unable to look after their children. However, not only have they been leaving their children unsupervised, but both children have poor school attendance. Susie's behaviour at school is also worrying, and may be a result of her challenging home life.

Case summary

There are multiple risk factors and concerning features in this case that should lead you to suspect neglect. These signs should not be ignored, and a social care referral should be made.

Case 9.3 Developmental delay

You are running a general paediatric outpatient clinic and see Priya, a three-year-old girl referred by her GP with concerns of developmental delay as she only has a few words and seems withdrawn. You start by trying to engage Priya in some games, but despite encouragement she seems very uninterested. She avoids eye contact and does not speak. When you ask her mother, Shanti, whether this is normal, she admits that Priya has very few words. You ask Shanti about her family situation, and she tells you that she rarely leaves the house and that her mother-in-law makes most of the decisions about Priya's care.

Case 9.3 Exercise

◆ Are there concerning features in the history?

◆ What further investigations would you want to do?

Case 9.3 Discussion

Are there concerning features in the history?

◆ Priya seems to have no expressive language—a potential outcome of neglect (Cantwell and Baker, 1985).

◆ Shanti sounds very socially isolated and uninvolved in her daughter's care. If Priya is being brought up in an environment where there is very little social interaction, her language development will be directly impacted.

◆ Priya could not be engaged in play. Considering the history it is possible that she has not been given opportunities to play at home. Play is vital for child development—not only does it help a child to learn motor skills but it is often the primary mode of communication between parent and child. Without it, a child misses out on opportunities to practise their social communication skills and development is affected.

◆ It is unclear whether Priya attends nursery, and if not she is missing out on another prime opportunity for these same skills to be developed outside the home.

What further investigations would you want to do?

◆ A full social history should be obtained, focusing on how the care of Priya is shared and what the home environment is like.

◆ A formal assessment of every aspect of Priya's development would need to be carried out to see if there is delay in any other areas. The Griffiths Scales of Mental Development would be a possible tool for assessment.

◆ A hearing screen should also be done, and if normal Priya should be assessed to determine whether there are any other features suggesting autism or learning difficulties as a cause of her language problems.

Case summary

Being brought up in an environment that has very little sensory stimulation or opportunity for social interaction can be very detrimental to a child's development, and can constitute neglect if deemed to be severe enough.

Conclusion

Neglect can present in many ways and can be hard to detect from a single inter-action with a child and family. Sometimes a picture has to be pieced together from many interactions in many situations, which is why 'working together' between health professionals and their partner agencies is so important.

References

Cantwell, D.P., Baker, L. (1985). Psychiatric and learning disorders in children with speech and language disorders: A descriptive analysis. *Advances in Learning and Behavioral Disabilities*, **4**, 29–47.

Children and Young Persons Act 1933 (c.12). London: HMSO.

Department for Education. (2013). *Characteristics of Children in Need in England, 2012–2013. Statistical First Release*. Available at: https://www.gov.uk/government/uploads/system/uploads/attachment_data/file/254084/SFR45–2013_Text.pdf (accessed 14 January 2014).

NICE (National Institute for Health and Care Excellence). (2009*). When to Suspect Child Maltreatment*. Available at: http://www.nice.org.uk/guidance/cg89/resources/guidance-when-to-suspect-child-maltreatment-pdf (accessed 8 March 2015).

Radford, L., Corral, S., Bradley, C., et al. (2011). *Child Abuse and Neglect in the UK Today*. London: NSPCC. Available at: http://www.nspcc.org.uk/Inform/research/findings/child_abuse_neglect_research_PDF_wdf84181.pdf (accessed 7 October 2014).

10

Other types of abuse

Katherine Taylor and Gayle Hann

Chapter summary

This chapter covers complex types of abuse which often have an insidious onset, such as fabricated or induced illness and neglect of medical needs in childhood which can often overlap with psychosomatic and hysterical disorders. Childhood obesity, which is not only a public health issue but may constitute harm, is also covered.

Case 10.1 Apnoeas

Sophie, a four-month-old baby, presents for the eighth time to the emergency department with an apnoeic episode, with a background of crying and unsettledness. Her mother, Daniella, reports that she fed her half an hour before taking her out. Daniella says that, whilst out, she noticed that Sophie had turned blue. She picked her up and patted her on the back and soon Sophie returned to a normal colour. Daniella is concerned as this has happened many times.

Sophie was born at term weighing 3.69 kg. She has had numerous investigations including a pH study, an EEG, an ECG, a chest X-ray, and an echocardiogram, and she is awaiting an MRI scan. All tests have been normal. She has been admitted overnight three times and had a normal examination with no further apnoeas on each occasion. Her GP started her on domperidone and ranitidine a month ago as he believed she had gastro-oesophageal reflux. After seeing an allergy specialist privately, Sophie was started on neocate for cow's milk protein intolerance. Daniella reports that there has been no change in either the crying or unsettledness despite these interventions.

You examine Sophie and she is alert and smiling with a normal examination. You notice that Daniella is easily reassured but seems reluctant for Sophie to be discharged. She keeps asking if the MRI could be done urgently and wants repeat blood tests. She cannot understand why doctors keep sending Sophie home. She becomes defensive when you start asking for a social history, saying that you are not taking her seriously.

Case 10.1 Exercise

◆ What would make you consider fabricated or induced illness in this case?

◆ What is fabricated or induced illness?

◆ What are the features of fabricated or induced illness?

◆ How can you take this further?

Case 10.1 Discussion

What would make you consider fabricated or induced illness in this case?

Sophie has had multiple presentations to different health professionals but no abnormal findings either on examination or investigation. Her reported apnoeas are concerning but are not supported by an underlying diagnosis. Daniella appears easily reassured yet asks for more tests as well as becoming defensive when a social history is taken.

What is fabricated or induced illness?

Fabricated or induced illness is the current term for what was previously referred to as 'Munchausen syndrome by proxy'; another term is 'child abuse in the medical setting' (Bass and Glaser, 2014). Fabricated or induced illness describes a behaviour pattern where parents or caregivers exaggerate, induce, or fabricate physical and mental health problems in children in order to mislead medical services, the process of which places the child at risk of serious harm (Flaherty et al., 2013). In clinical practice it can be difficult to distinguish fabricated or induced illness from the concerns of those parents who are genuinely anxious about their child's well-being but have a distorted view of their health needs. However, it is important to maintain a high index of suspicion, as significant physical, emotional, and behavioural morbidity is associated with this form of abuse.

An incidence of 0.5–2.0 per 100,000 children under 16 years has been reported (Bass and Glaser, 2014), with a significant number experiencing major physical illness (RCPCH, 2009) and mortality rates estimated as 6–9 per cent. It affects boys and girls equally, and is not limited to any particular country, social class, or ethnic group.

What are the features of fabricated or induced illness?

It may present as verbal fabrication of symptoms or signs in the child (pain, seizures, vomiting, diarrhoea, or blood loss), or actual falsification of signs (putting blood in nappies, adding glucose to urine samples, applying substances to the skin to cause a rash). It can extend to withholding medication to induce physical signs (not giving midazolam to terminate seizures, or not giving insulin to a diabetic patient), or poisoning with medications or other agents to cause illness (salt, bleach, faeces). It can also include inducing apnoea or seizures, or fatal smothering).

There are many situations where you may begin to suspect fabricated or induced illness:

◆ reported symptoms that are not consistent with any known medical diagnosis

◆ unexplained poor response of medical problems to treatment or interventions, or an unexpected deterioration in a patient's clinical condition

◆ signs and symptoms that do not occur in the carer's absence, or when hospital staff are solely responsible for caregiving

◆ reporting of new symptoms as soon as previous problems have resolved, or multiple unconnected symptoms

◆ significant limitation of child's activities and daily living beyond what would reasonably be expected with the suspected disorder (e.g. limited school attendance, need for special aids)

◆ incongruous examination findings, or laboratory results which are inconsistent with the diagnosis or are clinically implausible

◆ presentation to numerous different health professionals inappropriately.

How can you take this further?

Any concerns should be raised with the lead consultant for child protection. The child's safety, and whether a planned admission would be necessary, should be considered. A chronology of events should be compiled, and a strategy meeting between the paediatrician, GP, school, and other agencies should take place if fabricated or induced illness is a possibility. A social care referral may be needed and specialist investigations, such as toxicology, forensic examination, or covert video surveillance, may need to be considered. The named doctor may even want to seek advice externally from the designated nurse or doctor.

Case 10.2 Developmental delay and recurrent illness

Danny, a ten-year-old boy with severe developmental delay, was admitted to your ward seven weeks ago with fever, drowsiness, and vomiting. He was commenced on intravenous antibiotics for suspected sepsis. He is exclusively gastrostomy fed and his mother, Cynthia, takes responsibility for his care on the ward, including administering medications via the gastrostomy tube. She is very reluctant to let the nursing staff access the gastrostomy tube as it was dislodged during his last admission. Danny initially showed a good response to treatment, but on day 15 of admission had another episode of vomiting and drowsiness. He was restarted on antibiotics and his condition improved. He remained in hospital whilst a new hoist was fitted at home. Three days before he was due again for discharge he became drowsy and tachycardic, and antibiotics were restarted. On reviewing his results you note that previous blood tests are within normal range and his blood cultures are all negative. One of the nurses has commented that Cynthia is unwilling to leave nursing staff alone with Danny, and that she seems to be very friendly with staff and other parents.

Case 10.2 Exercise

- What might make you consider fabricated and induced illness in this case?

- What are the explanations for fabricated and induced illness?

- What barriers might there be to reporting concerns about fabricated and induced illness?

Case 10.2 Discussion

What might make you consider fabricated and induced illness in this case?

Danny's illness is not responding to appropriate treatment as you would expect, and he is developing new unexplained symptoms. His blood results do not support a diagnosis of sepsis. In this case, you may begin to suspect that his mother is introducing other agents via the gastrostomy tube to induce nausea and drowsiness.

What are the explanations for fabricated or induced illness?

Possible explanations for this form of abuse are complex. In the majority of cases the perpetrator is the mother, and she may have a history of abuse, depression, somatization, or personality disorder. Motivations for the caregiver can include extreme anxiety, attention-seeking, material gain, or a need to maintain closeness with the child.

What barriers might there be to reported concerns about fabricated or induced illness?

Healthcare professionals may be concerned about missing a genuine disorder and want to rise to the challenge of making a complicated diagnosis. There is also considerable pressure from carers to investigate and treat, and a wish from doctors to avoid conflict and complaints against them. Suspecting fabricated or induced illness goes against what is normally expected in the doctor–carer–child relationship, and in paediatrics we rely on carers to give us a full history of events.

Discussion points

Diagnosing fabricated or induced illness is a complicated process which begins with a detailed history, and involves a thorough review of medical records and a multi-agency strategy meeting. The key is to document all conversations with caregivers or colleagues accurately. Cases 10.1 and 10.2 show how insidious this diagnosis can be in presentation and highlight the importance of a thorough and detailed medical and social history and liaison with other health professionals. If fabricated or induced illness is suspected, it is often best that a single consultant becomes the point of contact for the family and the medical decision-maker.

Case 10.3 Poorly controlled asthma

Sameena is a seven-year-old girl with asthma who is currently an inpatient following a severe attack. She has frequent emergency attendances with severe asthma exacerbations, and has been admitted to intensive care twice in the last year. Her medications include salbutamol and beclomethasone inhalers. At her last respiratory clinic appointment increasing her treatment because of poor asthma control was discussed. Her parents report that when she has an asthma attack they give the salbutamol inhaler but it makes no difference. On this occasion they reported giving ten puffs of salbutamol hourly for six hours before calling an ambulance, and that Sameena usually needs her inhaler up to four times a day. Looking through her medical records, you note that she often misses hospital appointments. Her GP informs you that Sameena has not collected a repeat prescription for over a year.

Case 10.3 Exercise

◆ When would you start to consider abuse in this case?

◆ What else could be considered a neglect of a child's medical needs?

Case 10.3 Discussion

When would you start to consider abuse in this case?

Neglect is covered in detail in Chapter 9, but this chapter will consider it in relation to specific medical conditions—it can be thought of as part of the spectrum
that encompasses fabricated or induced illness. The intention in these situations
may not necessarily be to deceive, but the result is the same—harm to the child
which can impact on school attendance and psychosocial development. Two
extremes should be considered (Godding and Kruth, 1991):

♦ Undertreatment with the caregiver not providing appropriate medication,
  resulting in worsening of the child's medical condition and repeated hospital admissions with invasive or aggressive treatment required.

♦ Overtreatment with exaggeration or falsification of symptoms, leading to
  avoidable investigations and hospital admissions, and caregivers manipulat-
  ing the system to gain access to unnecessary medications.

Sameena's asthma is not responding to appropriate treatment. Non-compliance
should be considered in any child who does not show the expected response to
treatment. In this case, if the family are deceitful about her inhaler use and are
deliberately not treating an asthma attack, it constitutes abuse.

What else could be considered a neglect of a child's medical needs?

Other situations to consider include:

♦ removing a child from hospital against medical advice

♦ failing to engage with medical services by not attending clinic appointments

♦ excessive demand for investigations or medication in an apparently well
  child.

Case 10.4 Obesity

George is a 13-year-old boy who is currently an inpatient on the orthopaedic
ward. He underwent fixation of a humeral shaft fracture which he sustained by
tripping over in the park. George has no other health concerns, but he weighs
95 kg at a height of 160 cm, giving a body mass index (BMI) of 37. The orthopaedic consultant is concerned that his weight has contributed to his injury, but
when you discuss this with his mother she become defensive and says that it is
just 'puppy fat' that will improve as he gets older.

Case 10.4 Exercise

◆ What is childhood obesity?

◆ How could you take this further?

◆ What other agencies could be involved?

Case 10.4 Discussion

What is childhood obesity?

Childhood obesity is defined as a BMI above the 98th centile for age and sex, and is calculated as (weight in kg)/(height in m)^2. Normal ranges will differ with age, and there are various medical, environmental, and social factors that can influence a child's weight and levels of activity; it is not always within the caregivers' control. However, it could be considered a form of neglect if weight concerns are not being addressed. There are extreme cases of children being taken into care because of concerns about their weight (Johnston, 2014).

How could you take this further?

You want George's parents to cooperate with the medical team if interventions and weight-loss strategies are going to work. Obesity is often a cultural problem and needs to be addressed in a multidisciplinary fashion. Explain to the parents why you are concerned about George's weight and discuss future health implications, and reassure them that support is there to help the family address his health issues.

What other agencies could be involved?

Physiotherapy, occupational therapy, and dieticians can all be involved during admission and can follow him up in the community, and the family can be directed to exercise and weight management groups. Social care does not need to be involved unless ongoing non-compliance and denial by parents leads to further medical problems impacting on long-term health.

Conclusion

Fabricated or induced illness, obesity, and neglect of a child's medical needs are complex forms of abuse and can present insidiously. Bass and Glaser (2014) describe a triangle of collusion between the child, the caregiver, and the health professional which occurs for fabricated or induced illness; the mother reports symptoms to doctors and may induce them in the child, while the doctors listen to the mother and at least initially collude with her by investigating and treating the child. Neglect of medical needs can overlap with fabricated or induced illness as well as neglect. Hospitals need to have a strict policy when a child is not brought for medical appointments in order to pick up this type of abuse. As health professionals, we are trained to listen to parents and trust that parents put their children's health first. In order to identify all types of abuse, we need to have a high index of suspicion and 'think the unthinkable', as well as having a thorough and structured approach to assessing the child.

References

Bass, C., Glaser, D. (2014). Early recognition and management of fabricated or induced illness in children. *Lancet*, **383**(9926), 1412–21.

Flaherty, E.G., MacMillan, H.L., et al. (2013). Caregiver-fabricated Illness in a child: a manifestation of child maltreatment. *Pediatrics*, **132**(3), 590–7.

Godding, V., Kruth, M. (1991). Compliance with treatment in asthma and Munchauen syndrome by proxy. *Archives of Disease in Childhood*, **66**(8), 965–70.

Johnston, I. (2014). Children taken into care for being too fat. *The Independent*. Available at: http://www.independent.co.uk/life-style/health-and-families/health-news/children-taken-into-care-for-being-too-fat-9158809.html (accessed 14 October 2014).

RCPCH (Royal College of Paediatrics and Child Health). (2009). *Fabricated or Induced Illness by Carers (FII): A Practical Guide for Paediatricians*. Available at: http://www.rcpch.ac.uk/system/files/protected/page/Fabricated%20or%20Induced%20Illness%20by%20Carers%20A%20Practical%20Guide%20for%20Paediatricians%202009_0.pdf (accessed 15 October 2014).

11

New challenges in child protection

David James and Sophie Khadr

Chapter summary

Safeguarding is constantly evolving. The exponential growth in communication worldwide has brought benefit to many people, but also brings new threats. The proliferation of social media and ready access to smartphones and the internet make it challenging to keep children and young people safe. This growth in communication has also increased the movement of people around the world. This sometimes happens against their will or under false pretences with a new life of abuse or domestic servitude. Gangs and gang-related violence also pose a significant challenge. We will explore these potential threats in five cases covering child exploitation, online bullying, trafficking, gangs, and radicalization, including the background to each problem and ways to help the young people involved.

Case 11.1 Grooming/sexual exploitation

Fifteen-year-old Anil presents to the sexual health clinic tearful and reluctant to talk. You explain his confidentiality rights and he begins to speak to you.

Anil is sexually attracted to men but feels unable to tell his parents or friends. Six months ago he visited an online chatroom for gay teenagers. He met Mark, who told him that he was 17 and had recently come out as gay to friends and family. They began chatting most nights, exchanged photographs, and arranged to meet. Before they met, Mark told Anil that he was actually 32 but that he loved him and age shouldn't matter. Anil was concerned, but met Mark for dinner, and over the weeks that followed they began a sexual relationship, often meeting at Mark's house.

Last night Anil was surprised to meet four men at Mark's house whom he did not know. Mark explained that they were friends who had seen Anil's photographs and thought he was good looking. One of them tried to kiss Anil and when he tried to leave the house Mark stopped him. Mark told Anil that if he did not cooperate, he would tell Anil's family about their relationship. Anil describes being held down while each of the four men raped him anally. No condoms were used and Anil is concerned that he may have caught HIV or another sexually transmitted infection.

Case 11.1 Exercise

- What should the doctor do now?

- What is grooming and child sexual exploitation?

- How common is it?

- What are the risk factors for grooming and child sexual exploitation?

- What are the signs of grooming?

- What support services are available for young people who are victims of grooming or child sexual exploitation?

Case 11.1 Discussion

What should the doctor do now?

Anil has been groomed and sexually exploited. He has also been raped (see Chapter 7 for more information on the treatment pathway for young people who have been sexually assaulted or raped). Anil should be directed to the local Sexual Assault Referral Centre for forensic examination and helped to inform the police. He should also be referred to a service for victims of child sexual exploitation.

What is grooming and child sexual exploitation?

Grooming is defined as befriending a child or young person and making an emotional connection in order to lower their inhibitions in preparation for sexual assault or exploitation. It may occur in person or online using social media or online gaming platforms.

Child sexual exploitation is sexual abuse of children and young people by those with power over them, often in exchange for accommodation, drugs, or gifts. There is natural progression from grooming to exploitation. Anil presented after the first instance of sexual contact with someone other than the groomer. However, by this time the groomer often has such power over the young person that it can be difficult to extricate them from the situation. Grooming often follows a pattern as shown in Figure 11.1.

How common is grooming and child sexual exploitation?

Exact numbers of victims are unknown. The UK Child Exploitation and Online Protection Centre received over 6000 reports of sexual exploitation in 2009–2010 (CEOP, 2011). Barnado's worked with over 1000 children and young people in 2012 because of sexual exploitation, and 413 children and young people contacted the UK's Childline in 2011–2012 (NSPCC/Childline 2012). However, this is almost certainly an underestimate. The insidious nature of the abuse means that victims may not recognize themselves as abused and abusers go to considerable lengths to avoid detection.

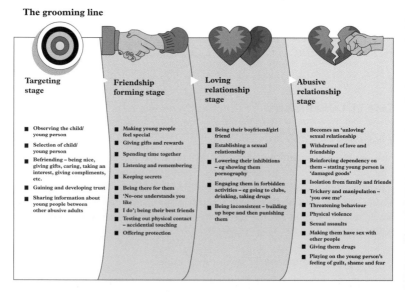

The grooming line

Targeting stage

- Observing the child/young person
- Selection of child/young person
- Befriending – being nice, giving gifts, caring, taking an interest, giving compliments, etc.
- Gaining and developing trust
- Sharing information about young people between other abusive adults

Friendship forming stage

- Making young people feel special
- Giving gifts and rewards
- Spending time together
- Listening and remembering
- Keeping secrets
- Being there for them
- 'No-one understands you like
- I do'; being their best friends
- Testing out physical contact – accidental touching
- Offering protection

Loving relationship stage

- Being their boyfriend/girl friend
- Establishing a sexual relationship
- Lowering their inhibitions – eg showing them pornography
- Engaging them in forbidden activities – eg going to clubs, drinking, taking drugs
- Being inconsistent – building up hope and then punishing them

Abusive relationship stage

- Becomes an 'unloving' sexual relationship
- Withdrawal of love and friendship
- Reinforcing dependency on them – stating young person is 'damaged goods'
- Isolation from family and friends
- Trickery and manipulation – 'you owe me'
- Threatening behaviour
- Physical violence
- Sexual assaults
- Making them have sex with other people
- Giving them drugs
- Playing on the young person's feeling of guilt, shame and fear

Figure 11.1 The Grooming Line (see also colour plate section).
Reproduced with permission from *Bwise2 Sexual Exploitation: A preventative education pack for use with 12 to 17-year-olds in pupil referral units, residential units and schools, England and Wales Edition*, Barnardo's, UK, Copyright © Barnardo's, 2007. All rights reserved.

What are the risk factors for grooming and child sexual exploitation?

Grooming affects young people of both sexes and from all backgrounds. However, certain factors (see Box 11.1) reduce a young person's resilience, increasing the risk of grooming beginning and progressing to sexual exploitation.

Box 11.1 Risk factors for grooming/child sexual exploitation

◆ History of sexual/physical/emotional abuse or neglect

◆ Young carers

◆ Low self-esteem/self-confidence

◆ Homelessness

◆ Looked-after child/care leaver

◆ Truancy

◆ Ethnic minority background

◆ Refugee or unaccompanied asylum seeker/trafficked

◆ Mental health condition

◆ Drug/alcohol use

◆ Learning difficulties and disabilities

◆ Gang involvement

What are the signs of grooming?

The signs can be subtle and include:

◆ unexplained behaviour changes

◆ inappropriate sexual behaviour

◆ disengagement from family or friends

◆ disengagement from school/truancy

- having unaffordable new things/receiving unexplained gifts

- multiple mobile phones/exaggerated anxiety around loss of phone

- repeated sexually transmitted infections/pregnancies

- involvement in crime

- self-harming/suicide attempt

- alcohol/drug use.

What support services are available for young people who are victims of grooming or child sexual exploitation?

Whilst a young person's physical health can suffer, the largest impact is on a victim's psychological health. They often need considerable help to exit the abusive situation and rebuild their lives. Young people must be managed by a multidisciplinary team with experience in supporting victims of sexual exploitation. This should include social care. A number of charities have considerable expertise and offer guidance and direct support for affected young people:

- http://www.barnados.org.uk

- http://www.nspcc.org.uk

- http://www.childrenssociety.org.uk

- http://www.paceuk.info

Case 11.2 Sexting and online bullying

Sixteen-year-old Katie presents to the Emergency Department after taking 14 paracetamol tablets. She wanted to 'fall asleep and not wake up'.

Katie discloses that she has been receiving abuse via Facebook since naked photographs of her appeared on the internet. Katie has been dating her boyfriend Chris, 15 years-old, for three months. One evening Chris asked Katie to send him a photo of her naked. She felt a bit nervous about this but complied. Soon afterwards, Katie began getting inappropriate comments at school and realized that other people had seen the photo. It was posted on Facebook and Twitter, and she began receiving messages from strangers including threats of sexual violence. She does not know what to do and cannot see a way out.

Case 11.2 Exercise

◆ What should the doctor do?

◆ What is sexting?

◆ Why do young people sext?

◆ Is sexting harmful?

◆ What is online bullying?

◆ What are Katie's options for resolving the problem?

Case 11.2 Discussion

What should the doctor do?

The doctor's first priority is Katie's immediate safety after her overdose. Katie is well with no evidence of a psychiatric disorder and blood paracetamol levels below the treatment threshold. She is assessed as low risk for further suicide attempts and just wants to resolve the bullying about the photo.

What is sexting?

Sexting is sending or receiving sexually explicit text, image, or video via mobile phone. This can be via text message, email, or chat functions on social media sites.

Why do young people sext?

There are many reasons why young people sext:

◆ feel in a loving relationship and enjoy it

◆ maintain or promote a sexual relationship despite living apart

◆ desire to show off their body

◆ perceived peer pressure

◆ pressure from partner

◆ desire to prove their sexuality or maturity.

Is sexting harmful?

Prevalence rates vary depending on the definition used. One large study suggests that 15 per cent of young people of secondary school age have actively engaged in sexting (Rice et al., 2012). Young people are more likely to be sexually active physically if they sext (Temple et al., 2012). Some argue that sexting represents a new step in adolescent sexuality and should now be classed as normal behaviour. However, young people often sext without knowledge of its potential consequences. Once a picture is sent, the sender no longer has control over it and it can spread quickly. This can lead to bullying, particularly online, or be used to facilitate sexual exploitation. The act of making and sending an explicit photo of a young person is illegal, as it is classed as an image of child abuse. There have been criminal cases in the UK, the USA, and Australia.

What is online bullying?

Online or cyber bullying is increasing in the UK and abroad. Recent research showed that up to 38 per cent of young people have experienced online bullying (NSPCC, 2013). It is more common among girls and disabled, homosexual, bisexual, or transgender adolescents. Online bullying can occur by text message, by email, or via social media sites. It can happen 24 hours a day and has been acknowledged as a contributing factor in several high-profile suicides involving young people.

What are Katie's options for resolving the problem?

Katie should be told that her situation is not unusual and that she is not to blame for what has happened. She also needs to know that there are a number of ways she can get help.

All the main social media sites have clear policies on bullying and harassment. Facebook has a button on its front screen which allows users to report inappropriate comments or photos. Twitter and other social media sites offer similar functions. Facebook also bans any nude photos. Young people may need help to navigate these websites to have content reported and removed.

Katie can report the cyber bullying to the police. Although there is no specific UK law on cyber bullying, there are a number of UK laws which can be used to prosecute, including the Protection from Harassment Act 1997, the Malicious Communications Act 1988, and the Defamation Act 2013.

Katie needs someone whom she can trust to talk to. This may be a parent, carer, or teacher. Childline offers one-to-one counselling online for young people who have been exposed to online bullying. She can access further support from organizations such as Childline, the National Society for the Prevention of Cruelty to Children, and Kidscape.

Case 11.3 Trafficking

Sixteen-year-old Fatima is brought to the Emergency Department by the police. She is shaken, thin, and has a headache. You meet her with an interpreter.

Fatima is Kosovan and her mother is widowed. Six months ago she met 20-year-old Artan in her home town in Kosovo and they began a relationship. Artan treated Fatima well, and she and her family were impressed by him. Artan had been living in the UK since adolescence. He told Fatima that he loved her and would bring her to the UK so that they could get married. He arranged fake papers for her and they travelled to the UK together four months ago.

Since her arrival, Fatima has been held captive in Artan's flat. He is physically and sexually violent towards her every day. Artan's mother lives with them and treats Fatima like a slave. This afternoon, Fatima escaped and ran to a passing traffic warden for help. The police have brought her to hospital because she disclosed that Artan raped her and beat her over the head earlier today.

Case 11.3 Exercise

- What are your priorities in assessing Fatima?

- What is child trafficking?

- What psychosocial and legal issues might Fatima face?

Case 11.3 Discussion

What are your priorities in assessing Fatima?

The first priority is to assess Fatima's head injury and any other injuries. She may be malnourished and at risk of refeeding syndrome. A menstrual and recent sexual history will help determine her risk of pregnancy. She may need a pregnancy test and emergency contraception. Once stable, you need to check that police have contacted a Sexual Assault Referral Centre to arrange a forensic examination and aftercare.

What is child trafficking?

The Palermo Protocol (UN, 2000), which is in force in the UK, defines child trafficking as the 'recruitment, transportation, transfer, harbouring or receipt' of someone aged under 18 for the purposes of exploitation. Children cannot consent to their own exploitation, even if they agree to being moved. Sexual exploitation and domestic servitude are among many recognized forms of exploitation; others include forced marriage, illegal adoption, organ removal, involvement in criminal activity, and use for labour, residency applications, or benefit fraud.

The secretive nature of child trafficking makes it is difficult to know its extent and scale. Victims may be trafficked into, around, or out of the UK. Traffickers target children who are vulnerable due to poverty, lack of education, limited job opportunities, or lack of family support. Victims frequently suffer multiple forms of abuse, neglect, and intimidation. Many are threatened with exposure to the authorities or violence towards family members if they try to escape. Most are aged 12 years or older when they are discovered.

The UK Human Trafficking Centre works to combat trafficking within the UK and internationally. Its partners include the police, the UK Border Agency, and non-governmental organizations including charities. Information sharing is facilitated through the National Referral Mechanism, a framework for identifying victims of human trafficking and ensuring that they receive appropriate care.

What psychosocial and legal issues might Fatima face?

Many victims of trafficking experience physical symptoms, mental health difficulties, or problems with substance misuse. They or family members may remain in danger even after their discovery. Multiple agencies are involved, and many victims find it difficult to know whom they can trust. They may be confused about entitlement to support, particularly if their age is in question. At worst, they could risk prosecution for criminal activity or deportation. Many victims go missing from local authority care.

Foreign victims of child trafficking have the same rights to protection and support as British children (DfE and Home Office, 2011). The Council of Europe Convention on Action against Trafficking in Human Beings (Council of Europe, 2005), ratified by the UK, additionally stipulates that where the age of a victim is unclear, he/she should be presumed to be a child pending verification of his/her age.

Further resources can be found at:

♦ http://www.nationalcrimeagency.gov.uk/about-us/what-we-do/specialist-capabilities/uk-human-trafficking-centre

♦ http://www.ecpat.org.uk/.

Case 11.4 Gang involvement and violence

Adrian, fifteen years old, has been admitted to the ward with a stab wound to the right shoulder. He tells police that he was stabbed by a stranger, but they suspect gang-related violence. Adrian lives with his mother and younger brother. He has a Supervision Order and a worker from the Youth Offending Team. Whilst in hospital, Adrian makes phone calls where he sounds agitated, and you are concerned that he may be at risk of further violence or an act of retribution.

Case 11.4 Exercise

◆ Describe some risk factors and concerning activities commonly associated with gang membership.

◆ How would you address your concerns about Adrian's behaviour and mechanism of injury?

◆ What other help can you offer Adrian?

Describe some risk factors and concerning activities commonly associated with gang membership

Risk factors and concerning activities are listed in Boxes 11.2 and 11.3, respectively.

Box 11.2 Risk factors for gang violence

◆ Male gender

◆ Childhood neglect and abuse

◆ Personality traits (e.g. hyperactivity/conduct disorder)

◆ Poor family functioning

◆ Domestic violence at home

◆ Delinquent peers and gang involvement

◆ Living in a high crime area

◆ Alcohol consumption

◆ Social inequality

Reproduced from M.A. Bellis, K. Hughes, C. Perkins, and A. Bennett, *Protecting People Promoting Health: A Public Health Approach to Violence Prevention for England*, Box 4.3, p. 29 © 2012, North West Public Health Observatory.

> **Box 11.3** Examples of activities commonly associated with gang violence
>
> ◆ Drug use/dealing
> ◆ Sexual violence
> ◆ Physical violence
> ◆ Knife crime/stabbings
> ◆ Access to other weapons
> ◆ Initiation rites
> ◆ Retaliatory violence
> ◆ Territorial violence
>
> Data from DfE and Home Office (2010).

How would you address your concerns about Adrian's behaviour and mechanism of injury?

Adrian should be offered the opportunity to discuss his mechanism of injury in private, ensuring that he is aware of confidentiality constraints beforehand. You should explain your concerns for his welfare and ask if he or a friend or family member remain in danger. Adrian may prefer to talk to another adult: a relative, community member or social worker. However, many young people will not disclose information for fear of reprisals by their own or rival gang members.

Social care can tell you if Adrian has a child protection plan and a referral is required regardless. The hospital child protection team and Adrian's allocated social worker or Youth Offending Team worker need to be involved in discharge planning. There needs to be agreement that Adrian is safe to go home and a follow-up plan should be in place before discharge.

What other help can you offer Adrian?

Adrian's admission provides an opportunity to address his wider health and psychosocial needs. You could offer him a sexual health screen, ask about drug and alcohol use, and refer him to substance misuse services if appropriate. He may have underlying mental health issues. You can ask Adrian and his mother about his school attendance and any perceived educational needs. He may have a learning disability that has not been detected or symptoms that suggest attention-deficit hyperactivity disorder. Social care often refers those involved in gang activity to youth services.

Case 11.5 Radicalization

Fourteen-year-old Omar is in the Emergency Department with his parents Mina and Jaffrey. They say that he is usually a quiet studious boy and is the youngest of five brothers. Lately he has been shouting passages from the Koran and will only wear white. His father reports that he has been very secretive, deleting his search history on his computer whenever he uses it.

Today, Mina became very concerned because Omar covered his room in white bed sheets and laid white paper down to walk to the bathroom. When she asked him what he was doing, he starting screaming about wanting to join his Islamic brotherhood and tried to set fire to his room. She called an ambulance when he would not calm down and the paramedics called the police.

The emergency doctor manages to carry out some basic blood tests and refers Omar to the paediatric team for possible mental health assessment. The paediatric registrar agrees and Omar is admitted for assessment. When he is discussed in the psychosocial meeting, the named nurse for child protection raises the possibility that Omar could have undergone radicalization.

Case 11.5 Exercise

♦ What is radicalization?

♦ Are there any specific characteristics that might help health professionals to identify children at risk of radicalization?

♦ Is there any guidance on what to do if an individual has become radicalized?

♦ What should you do next for Omar?

What is radicalization?

Radicalization is the process by which an individual comes to adopt increasingly political, social, or religious ideals and aspirations that reject contemporary ideas or freedom of choice. These ideals lead them to support terrorism and violent extremism, and may lead them to join terrorist groups.

Are there any specific characteristics that might help health professionals to identify children at risk of radicalization?

There is no obvious profile of a person likely to become involved in extremism or a single indicator of when someone might adopt violence in support of extremist ideas. Radicalization is different for every individual and can take place over an extended period or within a very short time frame. Association with adults who hold extremist views or take part in extremist activity is an obvious risk factor.

Is there any guidance on what to do if an individual has become radicalized?

The UK Government's *Prevent Strategy* (HM Government, 2011) was designed as a response to the ideological challenge of terrorism and those who promote terrorist views. It provides practical help to prevent people from being drawn into terrorism and ensure that they are given advice and support. It works with education, criminal justice, faith, charities, and health.

What should you do next for Omar?

Although it seems that Omar is suffering from a mental health problem, concerns have been raised about radicalization. You should ask Omar's parents about his mosque and whether it is the same one attended by the rest of the family. The concerns about radicalization should be passed on to the Child and Adolescent Mental Health Team and documented in a referral to social care. Most social care departments have a multi-agency referral process where all referrals are discussed. The police are part of this multi-agency referral hub and will have intelligence on local radical activity.

Conclusion

All healthcare professionals who care for young people need to keep abreast of modern issues facing young people in our communities. The key strand unifying the management of all these issues is the adoption of a non-judgemental patient-centred approach, whilst empowering and supporting the young person to escape from their abusive situation.

References

Bellis, A.M., Hughes, K., Perkins, C., Bennett, A. (2012). *Protecting People Promoting Health: A Public Health Approach to Violence Prevention for England.* Liverpool: Department of Health.

CEOP (Child Exploitation and Online Protection Centre). (2011). *Out of Mind, Out of Sight: Breaking Down The Barriers to Child Sexual Exploitation.* Available at: http://ceop.police.uk/ Documents/ceopdocs/ceop_thematic_assessment_executive_summary.pdf/ (accessed 11 October 2014).

Council of Europe. (2005) *Council of Europe Convention on Action Against Trafficking in Human Beings.* Available at: http://conventions.coe.int/Treaty/en/Treaties/Html/197.htm (accessed 11 October 2014).

DfE (Department for Education) and Home Office. (2010). *Safeguarding Children and Young People Who May Be Affected by Gang Activity.* Available at: https://www.gov.uk/government/ publications/safeguarding-children-and-young-people-who-may-be-affected-by-gang-activity (accessed 3 July 2015).

DfE (Department for Education) and Home Office. (2011). *Safeguarding Children Who May Have Been Trafficked: Practice Guidance.* Available at: https://www.gov.uk/government/ uploads/system/uploads/attachment_data/file/177033/DFE-00084–2011.pdf (accessed 11 October 2014).

HM Government. (2011). *Prevent Strategy*. Available at: https://www.gov.uk/government/uploads/system/uploads/attachment_data/file/97976/prevent-strategy-review.pdf (accessed 11 October 2014).

Kork, L., King S., Ogilvy-Webb, K., Barnes K. (2010). *Bwise 2 Sexual Exploitation: A Preventative Education Pack for Use with 12 to 17 Year Olds in Pupil Referral Units, Residential Units and Schools. England and Wales Edition*. Ilford: Barnado's. Available at: http://webfronter.com/hounslow/learningtorespect/menu0/Child_protection/BWise2Sexual_Exploitation/images/Bwise2_Sexual_Exploitation.pdf (accessed 24 March 2015).

NSPCC (National Society for the Prevention of Cruelty to Children). (2013). *Statistics on Bullying*. Available at: http://www.nspcc.org.uk/inform/resourcesforprofessionals/bullying/bullying_statistics_wda85732.html (accessed 28 December 2013).

NSPCC (National Society for the Prevention of Cruelty to Children/Childline). (2012). *Caught in a Trap; The Impact of Grooming in 2012*. Available at: https://www.nspcc.org.uk/news-and-views/our-news/nspcc-news/12-1-12-grooming-report/caught-in-a-trap-pdf_wdf92793.pdf/ (accessed 11 October 2014).

Rice, E., Rhoades, H., Winetrobe, H., et al. (2012). Sexually explicit cell phone messaging associated with sexual risk among adolescents. *Pediatrics*, **130**(4),667–73.

Temple, J.R., Paul, J.A., Van den Berg, P., Le, V.D., McElhany, A., Temple B.W. (2012). Teen sexting and its association with sexual behaviors. *Archives of Pediatric & Adolescent Medicine*, **166**(9), 828–33.

UN (United Nations). (2000). *Protocol to Prevent, Suppress and Punish Trafficking in Persons, Especially Women and Children, Supplementing the UN Convention on Transnational Organised Crime (the Palermo Protocol)*. Available at: http://www.uncjin.org/Documents/Conventions/dcatoc/final_documents_2/convention_%20traff_eng.pdf (accessed 11 October 2014).

12

Child maltreatment and cultural competence

Christopher Hands

Chapter summary

UK society is highly diverse, providing a home to people from a wide variety of cultural, linguistic, and religious traditions. Occasionally safeguarding issues and child protection concerns arise in the context of culture or migration which can make it difficult to identify how best to uphold a child's rights. This chapter addresses some of the most important instances in which a child's or family's national or cultural background may influence the well-being of a child in your care.

Case 12.1 Corporal punishment

You see seven-year-old Modibo in the Emergency Department. He is from Guinea and has come to hospital from school, accompanied by his father and a social worker, after his teacher noticed a cut on his face. The social worker explains that Modibo's teacher became concerned when she asked him about the injury and he did not answer her.

You see that Modibo has a 5 cm straight-edged laceration on his right cheek. When you ask him about how he received the cut, he tells you that 'a cat scratched me.' Modibo appears anxious and looks down at the floor throughout the consultation. When you ask Modibo's father about the cut, he seems to look past you as he explains that he hit Modibo with a belt. It becomes clear that he struck Modibo with the metal end of the belt. He explains, 'Children must learn to respect their parents. It is part of our culture to beat them when they misbehave.'

When you ask more about the social history, you discover that Modibo's father sought asylum in the UK three years ago after fleeing persecution by the military government in Guinea. When he was granted leave to remain, he applied for Modibo to join him. He has two jobs, and is supporting his new wife and their two-month-old twins as well as Modibo.

Case 12.1 Exercise

♦ How might a family's cultural background influence your decision-making in safeguarding cases?

♦ How might Modibo's experiences have influenced his behaviour at home?

♦ How might his father's experience of forced migration have affected his mental health and his behaviour towards Modibo?

♦ What support is available to Modibo's father?

♦ What rights to NHS care do refugees and asylum-seekers have?

Case 12.1 Discussion

How might a family's cultural background influence your decision-making in safeguarding cases?

People with different cultural heritages have different attitudes towards corporal punishment and its acceptability. Parents may argue that corporal punishment forms part of their heritage and cultural practices, and it is important to counter this argument. Physical abuse of children is illegal throughout the UK (see Chapter 2) regardless of a family's national or cultural background. As in other cases of physical abuse, its discovery should prompt a referral to children's social care and a detailed social history to delineate stressors that may have resulted in the abuse.

How might Modibo's experiences have influenced his behaviour at home?

Modibo has moved from Guinea to the UK at a young age to live with a father he may not remember well and a stepmother he has never met. His father may not be able to spend time with Modibo because of his work commitments. Modibo is at high risk of experiencing attachment difficulties, and of displaying disruptive or aggressive behaviour, because of the early stresses he has experienced. Part of considering how to keep Modibo safe involves thinking about what extra social and psychological support he might need.

How might his father's experience of forced migration have affected his mental health and his behaviour towards Modibo?

Refugees are at increased risk of mental health problems related to experiences in their country of origin and on their journey, and experiences of adjustment after arriving in the UK (Craig, 2010). In particular, they are at higher risk of anxiety disorders and post-traumatic stress disorder. It is important to explore Mobido's father's current state of mind, and to discuss what support he may be able to access.

What support is available to Modibo's father?

Support for refugees who have experienced torture is available from organizations such as Freedom From Torture. Practical support is available from the Refugee Council and from refugee community organizations across the country.

What rights to NHS care do refugees and asylum-seekers have?

People seeking asylum in the UK, and those granted refugee status, have the same rights to NHS care as British citizens.

Case 12.2 A separated child from Eritrea

You see Haile, a 14-year-old boy from Eritrea in the Emergency Department. He has been admitted because of intractable abdominal pain and vomiting. Haile is lying in bed, but appears tall and very thin. He has been brought to hospital by a man who introduces himself as his uncle. It becomes clear that Haile speaks little English, and his uncle interprets for him, describing several weeks of abdominal pain and worsening vomiting. Haile does not look at you or his uncle during the consultation.

Haile has attended the Emergency Department twice already in the last ten days, and has been given omeprazole and anti-emetics. His uncle asks you for something to 'make the sickness stop'. When you ask about Haile's home circumstances, his uncle explains, 'He lives with me because he came here without his parents'. There seems to be no closeness or affection between Haile and his uncle. On leaving the cubicle, one of the nurses says, 'He should be moved out of the paediatric department; he doesn't look 14 at all'. You speak to Haile on his own, using a telephone interpreting service. Haile tells you that he is 13 or 14, that he came to the UK alone about a month ago, and that the man with him is not his uncle.

Case 12.2 Exercise

◆ Who is responsible for supporting separated children in the UK and what rights do they have?

◆ Where can you find guidance on working with separated children?

◆ What is the law on private fostering?

◆ What risks does Haile face?

◆ What challenges are posed by working with interpreters?

◆ How should Haile's age be assessed?

Case 12.2 Discussion

Who is responsible for supporting separated children in the UK and what rights do they have?

Children who arrive in the UK alone are looked after by children's services in the same way as other looked-after children, under Sections 17 and 20 of the Children Act 1989. Their rights are not affected by their immigration status as described in the Children Act 1989, 2004, and in the UN Convention on the Rights of the Child. This support is funded by the Home Office, although it does not necessarily cover all the associated costs. There are some differences between the arrangements made in the different countries of the UK; for example, in Scotland every separated child is allocated a dedicated guardian who is able to advocate for them.

Where can you find guidance on working with separated children?

The Separated Children in Europe Programme (SCEP) publishes a *Statement of Good Practice* (SCEP, 2010). SCEP is supported by UNHCR, UNICEF, and Save the Children, and offers clear guidelines on best practice.

What is the law on private fostering?

Private fostering occurs when a child under 16 (or under 18 if the child has a disability) is cared for and accommodated for 28 days or longer by someone other than a close relative, a guardian, or a person with parental responsibility. Close relatives are defined as parents, step-parents, siblings, siblings of a parent, and grandparents. An adult who does not have parental responsibility or is not a guardian or close relative, and who wishes to care for the child, must notify children's services of the private fostering arrangement. The law is defined by the Children Act 1989 and the Children and Private Arrangements for Fostering Regulations 2005. Terms such as 'aunt' and 'uncle' are often used loosely to describe extended kinship relationships, and may be used fraudulently to conceal the true nature of an abusive or exploitative relationship. Haile's revelation should prompt you to investigate further the precise nature of the relationship between him and his 'uncle'.

What risks does Haile face?

As Haile has arrived in the UK alone and is living with someone who is not an immediate family member, with whom he does not appear to be friendly, it is possible that he has been trafficked to the UK. If so, Haile is at high risk of being harmed or moved by his traffickers after his contact with health services. A referral to the National Referral Mechanism for trafficked children should be considered, as described in Chapter 11. Haile is at high risk of mental health problems as a result of his experiences in Eritrea, his journey to the UK, and his current situation. The majority of separated children are deported when they reach the age of 17½—some sources suggest as many as 94 per cent (Bhabha and Finch, 2006)—and anticipation of enforced return is likely to increase Haile's anxiety.

What challenges are posed by working with interpreters?

It can sometimes be difficult to be certain whether questions or responses are being translated accurately. Interpreters may come from the same region as a young person, but speak a different language. They may speak a different dialect of the same language; for example, speakers of Levantine and North African dialects of Arabic may not understand one another. Sometimes, an interpreter from the same region as the patient may have different sympathies in local conflicts or come from a different religious or cultural background. These factors may lead to the interpreter giving an inaccurate picture to either the doctor or the young person. If possible, it is helpful to double-check the child's understanding and level of comfort with the process regularly during the interview.

How should Haile's age be assessed?

Many of the young people who arrive in the UK alone are uncertain of their exact age. This can be because age is not commonly recorded in their country of origin, because of a lack of robust birth registration processes, or because documents have been lost in conflict or flight. Separated children may appear older than their chronological age as a result of their experiences of dispossession, flight, and survival in difficult circumstances. These factors can lead to children being disbelieved about their age. Where a child's age is disputed, children's services carry out a detailed age assessment; the child has the right to challenge this assessment if they feel it has not been carried out accurately. The paediatrician is an advocate for the child; it is not part of your role to carry out age assessments.

Case 12.3 Female genital mutilation

Five-year-old Ayaan has been referred to the community paediatric clinic after concerns at school about speech delay, fine motor delay, and disruptive behaviour in class. She is one of seven Somali children being looked after by their mother. You spend some time building a rapport with Ayaan's mother, who has attended with her 15-year-old daughter Aisha who is interpreting for her. The home situation seems chaotic, and Ayaan's mother explains that she is struggling to cope. After the family has left the clinic room, Aisha comes back in and tells you that she is very worried. Her mother is taking them back to Somalia this summer, and she is going to 'have the girls cut'.

Case 12.3 Exercise

- What is female genital mutilation?

- What are the health consequences of female genital mutilation?

- What is the law in relation to female genital mutilation?

- What should you tell Ayaan's mother?

Case 12.3 Discussion

What is female genital mutilation?

Female genital mutilation is thought to affect 100–140 million women worldwide (WHO, 2012). The term describes a range of procedures, often involving partial or total excision of the external female genitalia, which are carried out for non-medical reasons (see Box 12.1) (Simpson et al., 2012).

What are the health consequences of female genital mutilation?

The health consequences of female genital mutilation may include pain, excessive bleeding, infection, keloid scarring, problems passing urine and stool, dyspareunia, and in some cases death due to uncontrolled haemorrhage. Some women who have undergone female genital mutilation experience long-term mental health sequelae, including post-traumatic stress disorder, depression, and anxiety.

Box 12.1 Classification of female genital mutilation

Type 1 Partial or total removal of the clitoris or prepuce, or both

Type 2 Partial or total removal of the clitoris and the labia minora, with or without excision of the labia majora

Type 3 (Infibulation) Narrowing of the vaginal orifice with creation of a covering seal by cutting and opposing the labia minora or majora (or both), with or without excision of the clitoris

Type 4 All other harmful procedures to the female genitalia for non-medical purposes—for example, pricking, piercing, or cutting

Reproduced from *The British Medical Journal*, J. Simpson, K. Robinson, S.M. Creighton, and D. Hodes, Female genital mutilation: the role of health professionals in prevention, assessment, and management, 344, e1361, Box 1, Copyright © 2012, BMJ Publishing Group Ltd With permission from BMJ Publishing Group Ltd.

What is the law in relation to female genital mutilation?

Female genital mutilation is prohibited under the Female Circumcision Prohibition Act 1985. Any person who performs, aids, abets, counsels, or procures an act of female genital mutilation is liable to prosecution. In 2003 the law was amended so that any person who performs, aids, abets, counsels, or procures female genital mutilation on a UK national outside the UK is also liable to prosecution.

What should you tell Ayaan's mother?

You must explain the health consequences of female genital mutilation to Ayaan's mother, and tell her that if she has it performed on her children she will be breaking the law. It may be difficult to influence her perspective in a short clinic consultation, and you should also make a referral to social care who will involve the police if the children are at risk. It may also be possible to refer to a community advocate to work with Ayaan's mother. Female genital mutilation is a harmful cultural practice that is not mandated by Islam or any other religion, and there is no justification for carrying it out or for allowing it to happen.

Case 12.4 Abuse linked to faith or belief

Maya is a six-year-old Congolese girl with epilepsy who is on the ward following a prolonged seizure at home. She was prescribed regular sodium valproate six months ago, but when you call her GP it transpires that her prescriptions have not been collected. When you examine Maya, you find several irregularly shaped scars on her back. When you ask her mother how she is managing Maya's epilepsy, she tells you that she is 'trying to get rid of the curse'. When you ask about the scars on Maya's back, her mother says 'I am trying to help her'.

Case 12.4 Exercise

◆ How would you address Maya's treatment with her mother?

◆ What are the possible causes of the scars on Maya's back?

◆ What are the possible consequences of witchcraft branding?

◆ What practices are involved in 'deliverance' from 'evil spirits'?

Case 12.4 Discussion

How would you address Maya's treatment with her mother?

The way that Maya's mother describes her daughter's epilepsy is concerning, and it is important to explore her beliefs and who else has informed those beliefs. It is possible that friends, acquaintances, or members of her religious community have suggested ideas about the cause of Maya's epilepsy. In order to support Maya effectively, you need to understand this context as fully as possible.

What are the possible causes of the scars on Maya's back?

The scars could be the result of traditional treatments, rooted in Maya's family's country of origin, that are being practised in the UK. It may be that Maya's epilepsy has been interpreted as being due to spirit possession or witchcraft, and that the scars are the result of practices aimed at 'exorcising' the spirits. It is important to ask Maya's mother directly about this 'curse' and how she intends to treat it. Maya is at high risk of further serious physical abuse.

What are the possible consequences of witchcraft branding?

Amongst some religious communities, including Christian, Hindu, Muslim, and pagan communities, children suffering from common health conditions, such as epilepsy, enuresis, or speech delay, may be labelled as being 'possessed' by 'evil spirits' (Briggs et al., 2011). Different words may be used to describe the magic believed to be involved, including 'juju' (West Africa) and 'kindoki' (Central Africa). The children are at high risk of social ostracism. Such branding places them at higher risk of physical and emotional abuse from those close to them.

What practices are involved in 'deliverance' from 'evil spirits'?

Children accused of spirit possession may suffer psychological harm because they are singled out and identified as 'different' and 'bad'. They may be ostracized within their cultural or religious community or subjected to exorcism rituals carried out by persons claiming to have skills in this area. Such persons frequently charge for their services, and so encouraging witchcraft accusations may be a source of profit. Children accused of spirit possession may also be exposed to physical violence if they are accused of bringing misfortune upon a family or a neighbourhood (Department for Education, 2012).

Case 12.5 Honour-based violence

You see Sapna, a 16-year-old Bangladeshi girl admitted with persistent vomiting and collapse. She has a positive pregnancy test on urine dipstick. Sapna tells you that she didn't know that she was pregnant. She has been in a relationship for the last year but has not told her parents. Sapna looks terrified and asks you not to tell anyone about her pregnancy or her relationship. She says that if her family find out, they will have her killed.

Case 12.5 Exercise

◆ What is 'honour-based violence'?

◆ What steps can you take to protect Sapna?

Case 12.5 Discussion

What is 'honour-based violence'?

Women from some cultural or religious communities, particularly Middle Eastern or South Asian communities, may be threatened with violence or death if they have a romantic relationship with a man who has not been approved of by their family, or if they try to avoid an arranged marriage to someone they do not wish to marry ('forced marriage'). Police figures indicate that there were more than 2800 acts of honour-based violence in the UK in 2010 (IKWRO, 2011), though there may be significant under-reporting. Whilst Sapna's fear that her family will 'have her killed' may be an overstatement, it may also be a realistic assessment of a serious risk to her life.

What steps can you take to protect Sapna?

Members of the extended family may collaborate to inflict harm on Sapna. It is important to inform both social care and the police of her situation. A risk assessment will be made, and possibly a plan will be made to accommodate Sapna in a refuge where her identity can be protected.

Conclusion

Many different aspects of a child's journey to the UK, and their cultural or religious background, may influence their well-being. It is important to be aware of these different aspects of children's experiences, and to be alert to potential harms. Engaging with the child's parents and understanding their situation and their perspective is important, but addressing harmful practices which are claimed to be 'part of our culture' is not racist. Whilst the communication involved may be difficult, identifying and challenging abuse which the perpetrators attempt to explain by reference to 'culture' is essential in successfully upholding the rights of children in a multicultural society.

References

Bhabha, J., Finch, N. (2006). *Seeking Asylum Alone: Unaccompanied and Separated Children and Refugee Protection in the UK*. London: Green Court Chambers.

Briggs, S., Whittaker, A., Linford, H., Bryan, A., Ryan, E., Ludick, D. (2011). *Safeguarding Children's Rights: Exploring Issues of Witchcraft and Spirit Possession in London's African Communities*. Available at: http://www.trustforlondon.org.uk/wp-content/uploads/2013/11/Safeguarding-final-report.pdf (accessed 4 July 2015).

Craig, T. (2010). Mental distress and psychological interventions in refugee populations. In D. Bhugra, T. Craig, K. Bhui (eds), *Mental Health of Refugees and Asylum Seekers*, pp 1–60. Oxford: Oxford University Press.

Department for Education. (2012), *National Action Plan to Tackle Child Abuse Linked to Faith or Belief*. Available at: https://www.gov.uk/government/publications/national-action-plan-to-tackle-child-abuse-linked-to-faith-or-belief (accessed 10 April 2014).

IKWRO (Iranian and Kurdish Women's Rights Organisation). (2011). *Nearly 3000 Cases of 'Honour' Violence Every Year in the UK*. Available at: http://ikwro.org.uk/2011/12/nearly-3000-cases-of-honour-violence-every-year-in-the-uk (accessed 10 April 2014).

SEPCO (Separated Children in Europe). (2010). *Statement of Good Practice* (4th edn). Available at: http://www.refworld.org/pdfid/415450694.pdf (accessed 10 April 2014).

Simpson, J., Robinson, K., Creighton, S.M., Hodes, D. (2012). Female genital mutilation: the role of health professionals in prevention, assessment and management. *British Medical Journal*, **344**, e1361.

WHO (World Health Organisation). (2014). *Female Genital Mutilation*. Available at: http://www.who.int/mediacentre/factsheets/fs241/en/ (accessed 10 April 2014).

13

Child protection in primary care

Bryony Alderman

Chapter summary

Primary care is frequently the first point of contact for family healthcare. General practitioners (GPs) have a valuable insight into children and their families—a context that may not be so readily available elsewhere. Understanding children and their environment may help to identify vulnerable children as well as those already being maltreated. Despite such apparent advantages, GPs may also find themselves faced with complex confidentiality issues. Both victim and perpetrator are usually registered with the same practice, and such conflicts require a careful and tailored approach to achieve the optimum outcome for all involved.

Background

General practice is typically considered the 'front line' of medical care, and is often the first port of call for families with healthcare concerns. Almost every child in the UK is registered with a GP, and to find one who is not would be very unusual (RCGP/NSPCC, 2011). Such is the GP's importance that many hospitals will avoid discharging any child who is unregistered, as recommended in the Laming Report (2003) (discussed further in Chapters 1 and 17).

Traditionally, GPs treated members of the same family, establishing long-term relationships with many of their patients. This ideal is not always replicated in modern lives, where people move frequently and family members may live many miles apart. Assigning a single doctor to a family is often impractical given the high demand for appointments and rotation of GP trainees. Despite this, and additional challenges such as short consultation times, contact with primary care is often less transient than in other healthcare settings.

GPs and practice nurses, whether through their own consultations or discussion with colleagues, can place children in the context of the whole family. They know of other household members, of significant events in the family's past, and the well-being of siblings. Children are seen in primary care for a whole raft of reasons—routine appointments, vaccinations, or simply while accompanying a relative. A GP might never see the child at risk, but instead identify adult patients with issues such as substance misuse or mental health problems that may put children at risk. Thinking 'outside the consultation room' is essential.

Case 13.1 Vulnerable families

You are a GP registrar in a busy inner-city practice. Your next patient is Jessica, 24 years old, mother to seven-year-old Jake, four-year-old Ella, and 14-month-old Mia.

Jessica wants your advice because Jake has demonstrated some worrying behaviour at school. He sometimes refuses to take part in lessons, distracting other children or leaving the classroom completely. He has shown aggression to other pupils in the playground, something which is particularly concerning his teachers.

Your colleague recently treated Mia for a urine infection, and you know that she has missed appointments made for her with the local paediatrician. She first sat unaided at 11 months, is not yet walking, and has no recognizable words.

Jessica does not work and lives with her children in a three-bedroomed flat; she has no other family nearby. She occasionally sees the father of her children but he was abusive to her in the past. Jessica says that she feels unsafe in her local area because there is a lot of crime and drug use, which makes her reluctant to leave the house.

Case 13.1 Exercise

◆ Are there any risk factors for child abuse?

◆ What are your concerns and what further information might you like to know?

◆ Does any action need to be taken with regard to child protection?

◆ Where can GPs get advice?

Case 13.1 Discussion

Are there any risk factors for child abuse?

You have access to valuable medical and social information about this family. There is no proof that abuse has taken place, but certain features presented in the history, such as domestic violence, Jessica's young age, and lack of other support, suggest an increased risk of abuse. Other general indicators include:

♦ alcohol or substance misuse, or mental health disorder in a child's parents or carers

♦ previous maltreatment of children within the family

♦ children who are disabled, or have a long-term illness.

Although none of these factors confirm that abuse has taken place, they can be helpful in identifying vulnerable families (see also Chapter 5).

What are your concerns and what further information might you like to know?

♦ Jake's behavioural difficulties are the reason Jessica has consulted you, so you need to discuss them further. Changes in emotional and behavioural state for which there is no obvious explanation might lead you to consider abuse, but identifying these indicators is challenging since they may be subtle. A review of the behavioural consequences of child abuse identified a number of possible indicators of maltreatment, including changes in behaviour (Odhayani et al., 2013) (the impact of abuse is covered in Chapter 3). It would be helpful to explore Jake's behavioural issues further, asking the following questions:

○ How long has his behaviour caused concern?

○ Is there an obvious trigger for his behaviour change?

○ Is the poor behaviour demonstrated both at school and at home?

○ How does he usually perform academically? Have there been recent changes/inconsistencies?

♦ You should find out more about Jessica's abusive relationship. You need to know whether domestic violence is ongoing, and whether the children still have contact with their father.

♦ Mia was not brought to the last appointments with the paediatrician, so you can ask Jessica about this. Recent Royal College of General Practitioners

(RCGP) guidelines suggest that children who regularly fail to attend routine appointments should be followed up, even if they are not subject to a child protection plan (RCGP/NSPCC, 2011).

◆ Jessica evidently finds her current living conditions challenging and mentions a reluctance to leave the house. You might wish to explore how she goes about providing essentials for herself and the children, and how Jake and Ella get to and from school. The school can corroborate this information and their attendance rates.

◆ Aside from the history itself, a great deal can be gleaned from observation. Simple considerations, such as whether the children are appropriately dressed and clean, are helpful. Consistent failure to meet these standards could indicate maltreatment. The interaction within the family is more difficult to assess, but you might pick up on features which seem unusual. Neglectful parenting may manifest as hostility from the mother, with reduced responsiveness and less verbal interaction with the child (Bennett et al., 2006).

Does any action need to be taken with regard to child protection?

There is no solid evidence here to justify an immediate referral to social care. Recognizing the difference in approach to 'softer' signs, as opposed to more obvious indicators of abuse, is essential. Guidelines from the National Institute of Health and Clinical Excellence (NICE) recognize a spectrum from 'consider' abuse, where abuse is just one possible explanation for a presenting feature, through to 'suspect', where you have serious concerns about abuse but no proof (NICE, 2009).

In this case, you can certainly work towards building a more complete picture of the family's circumstances and then use this information to guide your decision-making. A more complete picture may be gained by the following actions:

◆ Talking to other colleagues in your practice about their interactions with the family and whether there have been missed appointments.

◆ Reviewing the notes of all the children to see whether child protection concerns have ever been raised, any of the children have been subject to a child protection plan, or there have been other presentations potentially related to maltreatment. Since there are no immediate concerns about serious child abuse, you need to seek Jessica's permission to do this. You might consider looking at Jessica's notes to establish more about her own health needs and childhood experiences.

◆ Asking the health visitor about the family. Health visitors see children under five years of age for their immunizations and health surveillance and may know Mia and Ella. Reports from home visits in particular could provide a better understanding of the circumstances. The Personal Child Health Record ('red book') is a key source of information about a child's previous health, development, and well-being (see Chapter 9, Figure 9.1, for an example of a growth chart from the 'red book').

◆ Contacting Mia's paediatrician to share information and find out if they have any concerns.

Arranging a professionals' meeting could provide a valuable forum for discussion of the case, allowing a collective decision to be made about whether the threshold for referral for a full child protection investigation has been met (see Chapter 16 for more on professionals' meetings).

A newer initiative, which may be beneficial in cases like these, is weekly GP-led multidisciplinary team teleconferencing. This approach helps to coordinate care and facilitate information sharing between primary, community, and hospital services. Children who might be at risk can be selected for discussion using different criteria, for example those who have exceeded a threshold number of Emergency Department attendances. Children with chronic conditions, such as asthma or diabetes, who have frequent emergency admissions might also benefit from discussion, as poor control and parents' failure to adhere to treatment regimes could be suspicious for neglect.

If the threshold for referral to children's social care is not met, you can still arrange to review the family at intervals or ask Jessica if she would consent to a referral to social care for 'children in need' (this is covered further in Chapter 16).

Where can GPs get advice?

You could seek further advice from the named GP for child protection in your practice, the named nurse or doctor at your local hospital, the designated doctor in the community, or national bodies such as the National Society for the Prevention of Cruelty to Children (NSPCC) or your defence organization. You can contact these parties for more general advice, which is helpful if you would like additional support but if there are no definite indicators of abuse, you may be reluctant to discuss specific confidential details.

Case 13.2 Physical injury: could this be sexual abuse?

You are a Foundation Year 2 Doctor in general practice. Your next patient is six-year-old Ivan, who is brought to the surgery by his mother. Ivan's mother says that she noticed testicular bruising when her son returned from playing at a friend's house and complained of pain and discomfort in the genital region.

Case 13.2 Exercise

◆ How will you approach this case, or that of any child presenting with a genital injury? What features might you look for in the history?

◆ Will you examine Ivan?

Case 13.2 Discussion

How will you approach this case, or that of any child presenting with a genital injury? What features might you look for in the history? (See also Chapter 7.)

It is easy to assume that genital injuries are suspicious. Although sexual abuse is part of the differential diagnosis, there is still a great deal more information to be gathered and your actions will be strongly dictated by the history you obtain.

Accidental genital injuries do occur in children. The accident might have been witnessed and should have a history consistent with the examination. Mechanisms include straddle injuries from falling onto a bicycle crossbar, stretch injuries such as superficial lacerations of the perineal skin sustained when performing gymnastics, and falling forcibly onto objects (Kadish et al., 1998; Pierce and Robson 1993).

It is essential to ask both child and parent how the injury occurred. Since the boy was at a friend's house, it would be helpful to know who was looking after the children, and whether this person provided any explanation. If you are worried about ongoing abuse, you could ask whether the boy has complained of pain or discomfort before, if there have been any injuries, or whether there have been emotional or behavioural changes. Sexualized behaviours or inappropriate sexual knowledge in the context of genital injury would greatly increase the suspicion of abuse (see Chapter 7, Case 7.3). An unclear or implausible history of injury raises suspicion and may warrant referral. Any discrepancies in the history between a child and an adult, as well as any changes in the story, are concerning and need careful consideration.

Would you examine the child?

This question is also covered in Chapter 7. The decision to examine depends on the history. Although physical examination is a routine part of clinical assessment, intimate examinations of children need to be carried out with experience and sensitivity. If sexual abuse has recently taken place, clinical examination by a GP (or anyone else) could compromise vital forensic evidence. Guidance from the Faculty of Forensic and Legal Medicine of the Royal College of Paediatrics and Child Health (RCPCH, 2007) draws a clear distinction between paediatric forensic examination for witnessed or strongly suspected sexual abuse and paediatric examination performed for a perceived or actual medical problem where sexual abuse may feature as a differential diagnosis.

- If a clear disclosure of abuse is made or suspicion is high:

  - Do not examine the child, since specialist examination will be required by an appropriately skilled doctor with the expertise to record, interpret, and report the clinical findings, and liaise with other agencies to share this information.

  - Refer directly to children's social care, using any out-of-hours or emergency contact numbers where necessary. You can also involve the police, although this is usually the duty of the social worker who will directly involve the child abuse investigation team.

  - Explain to the child and family what you plan to do, and why, unless you feel that sharing this information might put the child at greater risk.

- Where there is no allegation of abuse, and suspicion is low:

  - You may examine the child to assess the extent of the injury. The key question to answer is whether the history you have collected provides an adequate explanation for the clinical findings.

  - Even if your suspicion of abuse is low, look out for worrying features such as bruising on the thighs, 'love-bites', and burns. Also be aware that a genitourinary examination performed in primary care has its limitations. Normal anatomical variation may be mistaken for abuse, and vice versa. Case series reviews have shown that the majority of children with a history of sexual abuse have a normal physical examination (Heger et al., 2002).

The presence of injury seems obvious as a potential indicator. Repeated presentation to the Emergency Department is a well-recognized alarm sign, and while GPs should be notified about their patients' emergency attendances or hospital admissions, the GP could be the first person to examine the injured child. A child who presents late, with an injury that almost certainly warranted immediate emergency attention, should ring alarm bells (NSPCC, 2010). The facility in primary care to look back over a child's history and appreciate home and family circumstances will help in assessing the scenario.

Case 13.3 Emotional abuse

A 28-year-old man, Mike, comes to your surgery following a recent sports injury. His seven-year-old son, Jonnie, has accompanied him to the appointment. Whilst you are examining Mike, Jonnie starts to play with the toys in your consultation room but becomes frustrated on finding that one of the toy cars is broken. Mike is dismissive when Jonnie shows him the toy, telling him to 'Shut up and sit down, I'm talking to the doctor.'

As they leave the consultation, Jonnie trips and falls in the corridor. You hear his father swear and berate him: 'I haven't got time for this! I'm already late for work. Do you want me kicked out of my job? Shall I tell them it's your fault?'

Case 13.3 Exercise

♦ What are your concerns?

♦ What are the difficulties that GPs might encounter with such cases?

♦ How would you proceed?

Case 13.3 Discussion

What are your concerns?

This case emphasizes the value of observation in primary care, and the opportunities to identify worrying features even if the child is not the focus of the consultation. Mike belittles Jonnie for 'indiscretions' which would ordinarily be considered innocuous, and shows him little warmth or attention. These may be features of emotional abuse.

However, this remains a difficult scenario, with no concrete indicators. Mike's dismissive and accusatory verbal exchanges with his son would undoubtedly make observers feel uncomfortable, and it is these feelings that raise concern, rather than any identifiable physical sign. What is more, you have seen only a snapshot of the interaction between father and son, and this may not be representative of their usual relationship, so you need to tread carefully before jumping to any conclusions. Proving that emotional abuse has taken place presents a challenge in general practice. Even knock-on effects, such as problems at school, antisocial behaviour, or difficulties in forming relationships (RCPCH, 2013), do not prove maltreatment. In fact, some authors have argued that evidence of ill-treatment, and not just evidence of the resultant harm, is needed to confirm that abuse has taken place (Glaser, 2002).

What are the difficulties that GPs might encounter with such cases?

◆ Meeting the definition of emotional abuse is difficult clinically, since it indicates the presence of continued emotional maltreatment. Even though GPs may care for families over a long period of time, they may only witness isolated events that are insufficient to raise significant suspicion. Compounding this, the child and perpetrator may not be seen together on repeated occasions, making a pattern of behaviour even harder to identify.

◆ Individual perceptions may vary, and so the threshold for defining abuse is arbitrary. Which specific actions or attitudes are relevant for the child's development? If a child has experienced such treatment long term, they have nothing with which to draw comparison and may feel that their situation is normal.

How would you proceed?

At present, Jonnie does not require immediate protection. Colleagues within the practice might provide additional insight into his family life, including whether there are any environmental risk factors for child abuse, such as parental mental health concerns, substance misuse, or poverty. You might wish to look through Jonnie's records and establish his general well-being and whether there are any presentations suggestive of emotional abuse, such as recurrent abdominal pain (as described in Chapter 2, Case 2.1).

You might like to know whether other institutions such as school have ever raised concerns. Past risk factors, and the suggestion that these negative interactions occur in numerous environments, would increase the suspicion of ongoing emotional maltreatment. It is unlikely that you would want to challenge Mike there and then unless you were truly concerned that Jonnie was at immediate risk of harm. As always, more information will be valuable in guiding your next actions.

Conclusion

Unfortunately, work in child protection is overshadowed by uncertainty, since abuse is hidden away by both its victims and its perpetrators. A clinician's fears of the repercussions of an overzealous response need to be balanced against the consequences of failing to act. As the safety of the child is paramount, professional concerns must be followed through if their welfare is in doubt, regardless of the perceived subtlety of clinical signs. Careful information-gathering aids this process, and provides the detail needed to consider each case on its individual features.

This chapter has explored some of the ways that child abuse may present in primary care, although the spectrum of real-life cases is broad and complex. Child protection is often described as a jigsaw, and primary care is in an ideal position to draw its pieces together. This chapter has looked at the benefits of general practice in terms of understanding families, their interactions, and their circumstances, and having close links with colleagues from whom to seek opinion and advice. Child abuse may manifest in myriad ways, and acknowledging its continued prevalence is the first step to ensuring that it is given appropriate consideration as a differential diagnosis.

References

Bennett, D.S., Sullivan, M.W., Lewis, M. (2006). Relations of parental report and observation of parenting to maltreatment history. *Child Maltreatment*, **11**(1), 63–75.

Glaser, D. (2002). Emotional abuse and neglect (psychological maltreatment): a conceptual framework. *Child Abuse & Neglect*, **26**(6–7), 697–714.

Heger, A., Ticson, L., Velasquez, O., Bernier, R. (2002). Children referred for possible sexual abuse: medical findings in 2384 children. *Child Abuse & Neglect*, **26**(6–7), 645–59.

Kadish, H.A., Schunk, J.E., Britton, H. (1998). Pediatric male rectal and genital trauma: accidental and nonaccidental injuries. *Pediatric Emergency Care*, **14**(2), 95–8.

Laming Report. (2003). *The Victoria Climbié Inquiry. Report of an Inquiry by Lord Laming.* Available at: https://www.gov.uk/government/uploads/system/uploads/attachment_data/file/273183/5730.pdf (accessed 12 October 2014).

NICE (National Institute of Clinical Excellence). (2009). *When to Suspect Child Maltreatment.* Available at: http://www.nice.org.uk/CG89 (accessed 31 January 2014).

NSPCC (National Society for the Prevention of Cruelty to Children). (2010). *The definition and signs of child abuse.* Available at: http://www.durham.anglican.org/userfiles/file/Durham%20Website/Resources/Children%20and%20Young%20People/definitions_and_signs_of_child_abuse_pdf_wdf65412.pdf (accessed on 12/10/2014).

Odhayani, A.A., Watson, W.J., Watson, L. (2013). Behavioural consequences of child abuse. *Canadian Family Physician*, **59**(8), 831–6.

Pierce, A.M., Robson, W.J. (1993). Genital injury in girls—accidental or not? *Pediatric Surgery International*, **8**, 239–43.

RCGP/NSPCC (Royal College of General Practitioners/National Society for the Prevention of Cruelty to Children). (2011). *Safeguarding Children and Young People: A Toolkit for General Practice 2011.* Available at: http://www.rcgp.org.uk/~/media/Files/CIRC/Safeguarding%20Children%20Module%20One/Safeguarding-Children-and-Young-People-Toolkit.ashx (accessed 11 October 2014).

RCPCH (Royal College of Paediatrics and Child Health). (2007). *Guidelines on Paediatric Forensic Examinations in Relation to Possible Child Sexual Abuse.* Available at: http://www.rcpch.ac.uk/system/files/protected/page/Guidance%20Forensic%20Exam%20Relation%20to%20Child%20Sexual%20Abuse.pdf.pdf (accessed 12 October 2014).

RCPCH (Royal College of Paediatrics and Child Health). (2013). *Child Protection Companion* (2nd edn). Available at: http://www.rcpch.ac.uk/index.php?q=child-protection-companion (accessed 12 October 2014).

14

Acute presentations: child protection in the Emergency Department

Jacqueline Le Geyt and Gayle Hann

Chapter summary

Many children, especially those who are being abused or neglected, have very little contact with medical professionals. A presentation to the Emergency Department (ED) will often be one of the few times that a child will interact with a doctor. It is estimated that 2–10 per cent of children presenting to EDs in the USA are the victims of either neglect or abuse (Leetch and Woolridge, 2013). With this knowledge in mind, the importance of vigilance and opportunistic screening for potential maltreatment becomes apparent.

Recognizing potential abuse can save a child's life or prevent a lifetime of suffering. Identifying abuse must take the same priority as diagnosing a life-threatening medical condition. Unfortunately, in practice the possibility of abuse, either as the cause of the presenting problem, or present in the background of the child's life, is often overlooked or missed. This chapter aims to be a guide for emergency doctors who work with both adults and children.

Case 14.1 A baby with a fractured arm

You are a Foundation Year Two doctor seeing Holly, a four-month-old girl, brought in by her mother, Joanne. Holly has been crying more than usual and not moving her right arm as much over the last few days. Her mother, Joanne, cannot think of any cause except an episode of crying whilst Holly was being strapped into her car seat a few days ago. On examination you find two small circular bruises over her right arm and think that her upper arm looks swollen. She cries when you try to palpate the arm, and has reduced movements. You request an X-ray. Holly's X-ray shows a spiral fracture of her humerus. As Holly is a non-mobile child, the presence of bruising means that non-accidental injury must be considered within the differential diagnoses.

Case 14.1 Exercise

♦ Is it likely that the injury occurred whilst Holly was being strapped into her car seat?

♦ Which injuries should worry us?

♦ What is the role of the emergency doctor in child protection?

♦ What should you do next?

Case 14.1 Discussion

Is it likely that the injury occurred whilst Holly was being strapped into her car seat?

At four months old, Holly would be unlikely to sustain a fracture easily unless there is an underlying bone disorder such as osteogenesis imperfecta. Being strapped into a car seat is unlikely to have caused such an injury unless done extremely roughly. She is also likely to have been in significant pain and would not have settled so easily.

Fractures in children aged under one year, particularly spiral fractures, should always raise questions of non-accidental injury. A systematic review demonstrated that the risk of a humeral fracture being abusive in a child less than three years was one in two, and a spiral fracture was the most common abusive fracture of the humerus in a child under 15 months of age (Kemp et al., 2008).

Which injuries should worry us? (See also Chapter 6)

Marks and bruises

♦ The developmental ability of the child must always be ascertained. Is the child mobile enough to have self-inflicted the injury as described?

♦ The location of the injury is also important; in mobile infants, accidental injuries and bruises to exposed areas such as the lower legs, arms, and head are more common, but less exposed or more sensitive areas such as the genitals, neck, ears, and oral frenulum are less likely to be accidental.

◆ The pattern of the bruise or mark should be looked at. Do the marks have the appearance of an implement? Are these circular marks around the arms, wrists, or ankles which could be signs of twisting or ligatures? Is it a bite mark? Or, as in the case of Holly, do they have the appearance of bruises caused by finger tips?

◆ Is the injury consistent with the mechanism given?

Fractures

◆ All fractures in a non-mobile child should be viewed with suspicion

◆ No fracture type on its own can distinguish abusive from non-abusive injury. Any fracture *could* be the result of abuse; however, there are some fracture patterns that should alert you to be more suspicious that abuse is a possible cause (Kemp et al., 2008):

  ○ multiple fractures

  ○ rib fractures, especially posterior or multiple rib fractures

  ○ mid-shaft fracture of the humerus

  ○ any humeral fracture in a child aged under three years

  ○ skull fracture in an infant or toddler

  ○ femoral fractures, especially in non-ambulant children.

What is your role as the emergency doctor in child protection?

◆ Your role as the emergency doctor is to *suspect* child abuse, to document history and findings accurately and impartially, and to escalate and report to the appropriate authorities. *It is not to confirm abuse.*

◆ You should ensure that you are adequately trained in child protection (see Chapter 21).

◆ commencing work, you should familiarize yourself with local child protection pathways. The majority of cases present out of normal working hours. *Know your local pathways.*

All EDs must be able to find out quickly whether a child is the subject of a child protection plan, or whether the child has recently presented to other EDs (RCPCH, 2014). The new Child Protection–Information Sharing project, a computer system that links the IT systems of the social care system with those of the healthcare system, will help with these recommendations.

What should you do next?

◆ You should document the exact wording of the history.

◆ Follow local protocols for raising child protection concerns—this will usually involve discussing the case with the paediatric registrar on call and making a social care referral. To do this you should have taken a family and social history which may have raised risk factors previously mentioned.

◆ Don't forget to give Holly some analgesia and refer her to orthopaedics, who will probably want to apply a cast or splint.

◆ Do a body map before the cast or splint is applied—a common mistake when dealing with injuries is to apply a cast without documenting bruising.

Case 14.2 A child with a burn

You are a middle-grade trust doctor in a busy ED in a district general hospital. Derek, 18-months-old, was brought in crying by the ambulance crew, accompanied by his mother Tanisha. She said that she had just finished ironing and left the room, and suddenly heard him cry. She found him next to the iron with a burn to his leg. She ran cold water on it and then called an ambulance. On examination, Derek has been screaming intermittently.

Case 14.2 Exercise

◆ What are your first priorities?

◆ What aspects are concerning about this case?

◆ What types of burns are concerning?

◆ What other presentations should worry you?

Case 14.2 Discussion:

What are your first priorities?

The first priority is Derek's medical care. He is screaming in pain, and needs analgesia and the burn to be assessed and dressed. Dressing often helps with pain as even air movement over a burn can be uncomfortable.

What aspects are concerning about this case?

Staff are unsure whether he could have caused such a burn accidentally because of its position. They also feel that, even if this has been an accident, Derek has not been supervised adequately. (Common places for accidental burns are covered in Chapter 6, Case 6.3).

What types of burns are concerning?

♦ Although both scalds and burns are common in mobile children, some particular burn patterns are suspicious for inflicted burns (see Chapter 6, Case 6.3). Dry contact burns showing the clear outline of an implement, such as the edge of an iron, as shown on Derek, or circular marks that could be cigarette stub marks, should raise suspicion. Scalds typically have splash marks without clearly demarcated edges.

♦ Some areas of the body are more suggestive of accidental burns or scalds, such as palms (grasping hot implements), head and neck, and trunk. Other areas are more likely to be non-accidental, such as buttocks, wrists and dorsum of the hands, feet, and legs (Hobbs, 1986).

What other presentations should worry you?

Inconsistent stories between caregivers and/or the child Suspicions should be raised if the details surrounding the injury or illness are inconsistent over time or between different carers. It is important to speak to the child separately, with an interpreter if necessary.

Injuries caused by lack of supervision Children of all ages have reduced danger awareness and it is the caregiver's responsibility to try to ensure their safety. Evidence of a lack of adequate supervision may be gleaned in the form of frequent repeated attendances for minor accidents. Was the parent was the influence of alcohol or drugs while looking after the child? Who was supervising the child? Did the parent leave the child in the care of an older but under-age sibling?

Incidental findings You should always be vigilant to the possibility of abuse, no matter what the presenting complaint to the ED. Ask yourself the following questions:

♦ Is the interaction between the parents and the child appropriate?

♦ Does the parent seem over- or under-anxious given the situation?

♦ Does the parent seem to have good parenting skills?

♦ Is the child's behaviour developmentally appropriate—or are there signs of the child being withdrawn, or interacting inappropriately with strangers?

Examining the child

◆ What is their overall appearance?

◆ Are they clean and well kempt?

◆ Do they appear well grown and nourished, or are there signs of failure to thrive or significant obesity?

◆ Are there any incidentally found injuries or marks on the body, and do these marks have appropriate explanations?

A number of centres have implemented screening questionnaires completed by the triage nurse or doctor, with many studies showing a significant increase in detection of abuse cases. An example is shown in Figure 14.1.

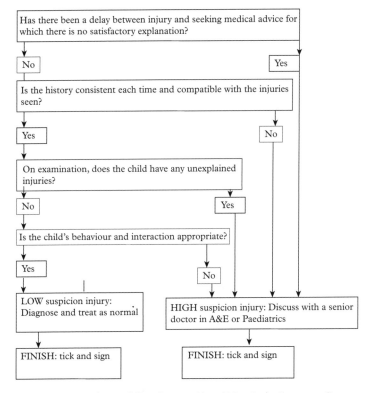

Figure 14.1 Assessing the possibility of non-accidental injury in the Emergency Department.

Case 14.3 Self-harm

Fourteen-year-old Zara presents for the sixth time with cut marks on her wrists following deliberate self-harm. While she was alone with the nurse who was cleaning her wounds, Zara broke down in tears and said that she did not want to go home. You are the emergency doctor who is asked by the nurse to see Zara. Zara confides in you that she does not want to go home as she is fed up with her parents pressuring her to do better in school. Tonight she reports that she cut herself after her mother asked her about the marks she had received for her English and Maths homework. Her mother called her lazy after she received B grades, saying that if she had worked harder she could have got As. She reports that she has taken an overdose of her mother's antidepressants in the past, but has not told anyone about it before. She also discloses that she is being bullied at school as she gets good grades.

Case 14.3 Exercise

◆ What are the links between deliberate self-harm and child abuse?

◆ Once Zara's cuts have been bandaged is there anything else you need to do?

Case 14.3 Discussion

What are the links between deliberate self-harm and child abuse?

◆ Deliberate self-harm can often be triggered by stressful life events or by more general feelings of distress that build up over time. Young people can use deliberate self-harm as a means of coping with emotional pain, or as a way of communicating their pain that they cannot otherwise express to others—a 'cry for help'.

◆ Child abuse, both physical and sexual, and witnessing domestic violence (see Case 14.5) have all been found to be important factors in self-harming by many children.

◆ Children who self-harm are much more likely to have concurrent mental health issues, such as depression, anxiety, and attention-deficit hyperactivity disorder, and be from deprived socio-economic backgrounds (Sidebotham and Heron, 2006).

Once Zara's cuts have been bandaged, is there anything else you need to do?

It is important to address the underlying causes of Zara's self-harming. Her stressors include parental pressure, emotional abuse, with her mother calling her 'lazy', and her mother's depression. You should discuss Zara with the paediatrician on call who, depending on the child and adolescent mental health services available locally, may want to admit her for a mental health review. A social care referral may also need to be made if any further emotional abuse is disclosed to the child and adolescent mental health services.

Case 14.4 Parental substance misuse

You are an emergency doctor on night shift. Maria, 24 years old, was brought in by police after being found at 3 a.m. asleep on the pavement. She appeared to be heavily intoxicated and spent two hours in the ED on intravenous fluids before being declared medically fit to be discharged. She tells you that she feels much better now and really needs to get home to her family.

Case 14.4 Exercise

◆ Why should you be worried about child protection in this case?

◆ What other information do you need to obtain to determine if there are child protection concerns?

Case 14.4 Discussion

Why should you be worried about child protection in this case?

Unfortunately, research shows that, despite vigilance, training, and raised awareness, many cases of abuse go undiagnosed. One reason for this is that the children themselves may not be present. Doctors in the adult ED working with parents or other people caring for children should be aware of risk factors that would make children vulnerable to abuse.

There are three major risk factors in patients presenting to an adult ED which substantially increase the likelihood of a child in an adult's care being the subject of abuse or neglect:

◆ domestic violence

◆ substance or alcohol misuse

◆ presentation with a serious psychiatric disorder, such as a suicide attempt.

Having any of these three risk factors within the home gives a positive predictive value of 91 per cent for children being the victims of abuse (Diderich et al., 2013). These three factors have also been cited in serious case reviews and are known as the 'toxic trio' (see Chapter 22).

If any of these factors are elicited during a consultation, as in this case, you should always ask the patient if they have children. Advice or local support services should be offered. If you feel that the children are at possible risk, you have a duty of care to escalate your concerns although the children are not your direct patients.

What other information do you need to obtain to determine if there are child protection concerns?

You should ask Maria about her family, particularly the names and ages of her children and who is looking after them. She may have left very young children at home alone. You should ask more about her drinking and what precipitated her to become intoxicated, as there may be other stressors in her life, such as domestic violence or mental illness, that increase the risk of abuse to her children.

Case 14.5 Domestic violence and self-harm

You are a Foundation Year Two doctor seeing Miriam, 39 years old, who presents after taking sixteen 500 mg paracetamol tablets. She reports that she took them after a fight with her husband, Ahmed, as he had been gambling and had lost their rent money. You note that she has had previous attendances in the last year for facial bruising and a broken wrist, and she admits that these injuries were inflicted by her husband. They have three children: 11-year-old Huda, nine-year-old Amina, and five-year-old Iqbal. She says that her husband has never hit her in front of the children and has never been violent towards the children.

Case 14.5 Exercise

- What is the impact of domestic violence on the children in this family?

- What should you do for the children in this family?

Case 14.5 Discussion

What is the impact of domestic violence on the children in this family?

The impact of domestic violence is greatly underestimated. The 2011–2012 Crime Survey for England and Wales reported two million victims of domestic abuse, with no significant change in numbers over the previous ten years (Office for National Statistics, 2013). Seven per cent of women and five per cent of men were estimated to have experienced domestic abuse. However, the abuse experienced by women is much more violent, resulting in more significant injuries and death. Two women are killed every week in England and Wales as a result of domestic violence (Smith et al., 2010).

According to the Department of Health, at least 750,000 children witness domestic violence every year. In some cases, the children themselves will suffer physical or sexual abuse from the same perpetrator. As in Case 14.3, domestic violence has a great emotional impact on children and is now recognized as a cause of emotional abuse, sometimes resulting in a child protection plan.

What should you do for the children in this family?

You have a duty as an emergency doctor to protect these children by making a social care referral for emotional abuse even if, as Miriam states, they are not witnessing the violence directly.

Conclusion

Emergency doctors are often the first, and sometimes the only, doctors with the opportunity to recognize the signs of child abuse. The role of the emergency doctor is to suspect child abuse, to document history and findings accurately and impartially, and to escalate and report to the appropriate authorities. Even when seeing adult patients, the emergency doctor, like the general practitioner, must maintain the awareness that their patients may have children who are at risk of maltreatment and act to protect those children accordingly. Doctors must also bear in mind that, legally in the UK, you are a child up to 18 years of age and therefore they may be treating children even in the adult ED.

References

Diderich, H.M., Fekkes, M. Verkerk, P. H., et al. (2013). A new protocol for screening adults presenting with their own medical problems at the Emergency Department to identify children at risk for maltreatment. *Child Abuse & Neglect*, **37**(12), 1122–31.

Hobbs, C.J. (1986). When are burns not accidental? *Archives of Disease in Childhood*, **61**, 357–61.

Kemp, A.M., Dunstan, F., Harrison, S., et al. (2008). Patterns of skeletal fractures in child abuse: systematic review. *British Medical Journal*, **337**, a1518.

Leetch, A.N., Woolridge, D. (2013). Emergency department evaluation of child abuse. *Emergency Medicine Clinics of North America*, **31**(3), 853–73.

Office for National Statistics. (2013). Focus on Violent Crime and Sexual Offences, 2011–12. Available at: http://www.ons.gov.uk/ons/dcp171778_298904.pdf (accessed 18 October 2014).

RCPCH (Royal College of Paediatrics and Child Health). (2014). *Safeguarding children and young people: roles and competencies for health care staff.* Available at: http://www.rcpch.ac.uk/sites/default/files/page/Safeguarding%20Children%20-%20Roles%20and%20Competences%20for%20Healthcare%20Staff%20%2002%200%20%20%20%20(3)_0.pdf (accessed 7 July 2015).

Sidebotham, P., Heron, J. (2006). Child maltreatment in the 'children of the nineties': a cohort study of risk factors. *Child Abuse & Neglect*, **30**(5), 497–522.

Smith, K., Flatley, J., Coleman, K., Osborne, S., Kaiza, P., Roe, S. (2010). Homicides, Firearm Offences and Intimate Violence 2008/09. Supplementary Volume 2 to Crime in England and Wales 2008/09. Home Office Statistical Bulletin 01/10. Available at: http://webarchive.nationalarchives.gov.uk/20110218135832/rds.homeoffice.gov.uk/rds/pdfs10/hosb0110.pdf (accessed 7 July 2015).

15

Child protection medicals: assessing children in whom there are concerns about child maltreatment

Katherine Fawbert

Chapter summary

This chapter is aimed at doctors who care for children, in both the community and hospital settings, and aims to guide them through the process of assessing a child where there are concerns about maltreatment. How to assess the urgency of a child protection medical, taking a history and examination, and related consent issues are covered. The best approach to assessing a child when an 'achieving best evidence interview' is planned is also described.

Doctors working with children are often involved in performing a medical assessment of a child where there are concerns about maltreatment. This is also called a 'child protection medical', or a 'Section 47 medical', named after Section 47 of the Children Act 1989. A Section 47 investigation is commenced when there is reasonable cause to suspect that a child is suffering or likely to suffer significant harm (see Chapter 16). This paediatric assessment is a key part of the overall child protection investigation, and it is vital to have a thorough and structured approach to ensure accurate recording of safeguarding concerns (see Appendix 2 for the medical proforma which standardizes both the assessment and the medical report).

The purpose of the assessment is broad and should include an evaluation of the child's wider medical and psychological needs. Your role is also to assess the likelihood of abuse on the balance of probability. As the doctor performing and reporting the child protection medical, you will contribute to the overall multi-agency assessment.

Case 15.1 Child protection medical due to concerns of physical abuse

You are a paediatric registrar performing a child protection medical for two siblings: four-year-old Rosie and two-year-old Maria. Their social worker, Pauline Heaton, has informed you of ongoing domestic violence. There was a recent police report that the children's mother, Julia, had been punched by their father, Joe. Julia also disclosed that Joe has hit Rosie whilst she has been at work, but she does not have any concerns that Maria was harmed. Pauline reports that Rosie's nursery key worker said that she noticed linear bruising to Rosie's right arm and a slap mark to her buttocks when she was changing her in nursery yesterday. She made a referral to social care. An *achieving best evidence interview* (Ministry of Justice, 2011) is planned.

Case 15.1 Exercise

- When and where should you assess Rosie and Maria?

- Who should accompany the children?

- What information should you expect from the social worker?

- How do you approach consent?

- How should you best proceed in terms of taking the history?

- Does the planned achieving best evidence interview affect your approach?

Case 15.1 Discussion

When and where should you assess Rosie and Maria?

Ideally, any child should be assessed within an appropriate child-focused environment, but more importantly with adequate time and by appropriately trained staff.

The Royal College of Paediatrics and Child Health guidelines (RCPCH, 2013) are clear that in cases of physical abuse the medical assessment should occur within 24 hours, especially if a police investigation is under way or protection from harm is required. Where possible, this should occur within normal working hours.

Who should accompany the children?

Generally the parent or caregiver should attend the medical, but this is not always appropriate if the parent is the alleged perpetrator. It is good practice for a chaperone who is familiar with the procedure to be present to aid both child and family, and also to assist the examining doctor. This person is usually the social worker. An interpreter or signer may be required for the child or parent. If you are a trainee performing a child protection medical, your examination and documentation should be supervised by a consultant.

What information should you expect from the social worker?

Before you begin the assessment with the child, the social worker should brief you separately with a summary of the child protection concerns and any other relevant information.

How do you approach consent?

It is usually assumed that a child under 10 years old is unable to give consent whilst a child over 10 is, although children obviously differ developmentally. You need to explain to their mother, Julia, the purpose of the assessment: that you need to take a history and perform a thorough medical examination including measuring growth parameters, and that you will produce a report that will be shared with relevant agencies. If photographs are required specific consent must be obtained, and often the police will take photographs themselves as part of their evidence. Written consent should be obtained. Legally a child can give consent to treatment but cannot refuse it. It is good practice to gain consent or assent whatever the age of the child.

In this case Julia can give consent as she has parental responsibility, but this is not necessarily held by a parent. Those with parental responsibility may include the local authority if an Emergency Protection Order is in place or a potential adoptive parent, or may be shared with the local authority (Children Act 1989).

How should you best proceed in terms of taking the history?

This should be viewed as a similar process to history-taking in any other setting, but with particular focus on the social background and close attention to relevant risk factors. Where possible you should always speak to the child alone, as well as with an accompanying adult, if they are verbally capable enough.

Julia has experienced domestic violence and this is a known to be a form of emotional abuse in children (see Chapters 5 and 8). All household members and those who care for the children should be clearly documented. On discussion with Julia, you find out that Joe has a history of alcohol misuse and has been violent towards her for years, but this is the first time that he has injured one of the children.

Does the planned achieving best evidence interview affect your approach?

In all cases open questions such as 'what happened?' should be used and not closed leading questions such as 'did Daddy hit you?'. When transcribing your assessment, and later when writing your report, it is as important to record the questions asked as well as the response to them, ideally verbatim (this is highlighted in Chapter 16). Where it is likely that an achieving best evidence interview will occur, typically when there is a high probability that the case will become a criminal investigation, it is especially important that only open questions are used to interview children. An achieving best evidence interview aims to gain an accurate account of events, and is performed by specially trained individuals in interviewing children. There is a particular emphasis on eliciting the child's free narrative account about any potential abuse. An initial assessment may still be necessary to gain an understanding of the broad picture and to organize treatment and an initial plan.

You should record contemporaneous notes using a proforma if this is local policy (see Appendix 2). It is important to cover the points shown in Box 15.1.

Box 15.1 Important points to be elicited in history-taking in a child protection medical

◆ Birth history.

◆ Past medical history including regular medications, allergies, and immunization status. The 'red book' or local health surveillance database may provide useful information. This should also include details of any multidisciplinary input the child receives such as speech therapy or physiotherapy.

◆ Development history: especially relevant in assessing the likelihood of injuries in relationship to development stage.

◆ Enquiry into school attendance and behaviour, including any extra support required.

◆ Systemtic inquiry including bleeding tendencies, bowel, bladder, and genital symptoms, and skin diseases.

◆ Any concerns or changes in the child's behaviour or mood.

◆ A clear social history documenting the family tree, including parents' health, employment, any new partners or step-siblings of the parents, and contact arrangements if parents are estranged.

◆ Risk factors in the carers should be sought, such as domestic abuse, substance misuse, mental health, learning difficulties, personal abuse of carers themselves in the past, criminal history.

◆ Previous or current involvement of the child or family with children's social care.

Case 15.2 Examination of a child presenting with a burn

You are a paediatric trainee working in the Emergency Department and see Tommy, a two-year-old boy. His mother, Sarah, has brought him because he is wheezy. When you examine him you see a linear mark on the palm of his hand that looks like a burn. When you ask Sarah how he got this mark, she tells you it happened a week ago at nursery when he fell over onto a radiator. You telephone the nursery and speak to his key worker, who informs you that they have no knowledge of an accident. You discuss your concerns with the paediatric registrar who, in view of the injury and inconsistent history, supervises you in performing a child protection medical.

Case 15.2 Exercise

◆ As the doctor performing the child protection medical how will you approach this situation?

◆ What will your examination include?

Case 15.2 Discussion

As the doctor performing the child protection medical how will you approach this situation?

When you speak to Sarah and explain that the nursery have no record of an injury she becomes very tearful. She explains that she previously had a social worker when she was in care as a child and panicked. She tells you that a week ago she had left Tommy alone in the living room for a minute to answer the doorbell after she had just used her hair straighteners which she left on the floor. Tommy picked them up with his right hand and cried. Sarah ran back into the living room and soaked the burn with cold water; but did not think that it needed any more treatment.

In taking a history in cases of physical abuse it is imperative that you elicit the timing of the injury and preceding events, the explanations given, and by whom they are given. You should also clarify the actions taken by the parents or carer when the injury was discovered.

In this scenario, although there are concerns with respect to the initial reluctance to give the history and potential neglect, the eventual explanation is consistent with both the injury seen and Tommy's developmental capabilities.

What will your examination include?

You proceed to examine the child with Sarah's consent. An examination should document the following (see Appendix 2):

♦ The child's demeanour, behaviour, and interaction with their caregiver.

♦ The child's general physical appearance, including clothing.

♦ Measurement of growth parameters such as height, weight, and head circumference, including centiles and body mass index.

♦ A full examination which should include the mouth, behind the ears, buttocks, genitalia, anus, and soles of the feet (see the body maps in Appendix 6 with these areas drawn individually as they are often difficult to document).

♦ Any injuries should be documented with both a description and measurements and marked on a body map.

♦ The Tanner stage of sexual development in adolescents.

♦ In cases of suspected sexual abuse there should be a detailed genital and anal examination.

Case 15.3 Writing a medical report

You are the paediatric registrar in the Emergency Department and Stefan, a 12-year-old boy, has been brought in by his mother with physical injuries allegedly inflicted by his father. The triage nurse immediately asks you to review Stefan. You perform a child protection medical and then need to complete a medical report for the social worker.

Exercise 15.3

♦ Are there any tips on medical report writing?

♦ Are there any examples of or resources for how to write a medical report?

Discussion 15.3

Are there any tips on medical report writing?

Use both medical and lay terms in your medical report that so it can be understood by all. After your medical examination is complete you must communicate your findings as soon as possible. Sometimes a rapid response is required, and we advise giving the rapid report in the format suggested in Appendix 2 followed by the full report as shown in example here. You may also identify other medical problems that require further management and should provide a recommendation for appropriate actions depending on your concerns. The report should be checked, and amended where appropriate, by a senior colleague.

Are there any examples of or resources for how to write a medical report?

Example medical report

I, Dr Katherine Fawbert, qualified as a doctor in 2005, and have eight years of paediatric experience, completing my paediatric postgraduate examinations in 2009. I have the following qualifications: BSc (Hons), MBChB, and MRCPCH. I regularly deal with children where there are child protection concerns.

On 10 February 2014, I was working as a paediatric registrar in the Emergency Department of Greenslade Hospital. At 20:15 I reviewed Stefan Constantin, a 12-year-old boy, along with his mother, Maria and his sister, Lacrimoara. A paediatric nurse, Louise Jenkins, was present throughout the consultation.

Stefan was brought to Greenslade Hospital by his mother. I spoke to both Stefan and his mother separately, as well as together. Stefan explained to me that he had got into trouble at school as he had been rude to a teacher. Stefan's form tutor, Mr Parikh, contacted his father, Marius, by telephone to inform him that Stefan had a detention that evening. By the time Stefan came home from school his father was extremely angry, and Stefan told me that 'his father beat him'. He told me that his father whipped him with an electric cable multiple times. Maria, his mother, told me that she was very frightened and ran out of the house to her sister's house and called the police. Stefan's left thigh and left arm were particularly painful, and he was limping on his left leg.

Previous medical history Stefan has mild asthma and is up to date with his immunizations.

Family and social history Stefan was born in Romania and moved to the UK seven years ago with the rest of his family. The whole family speak good English. He lives with his father, Marius, 42 years old, and his mother, Maria,

41 years old, who are married. His parents own and work in a grocery shop, and they live in a flat above this. Stefan has a sister, Lacrimoara, who is five years old. Stefan is in Year 8 at Greenslade School. According to his mother it is unusual for him to be in trouble at school and he is academically able. Stefan denies any drug or alcohol use and there is no criminal history. Maria told me that her husband is sometimes violent towards her, especially if he has drunk too much alcohol. Marius has always drunk regularly, but recently he appears to have become dependent on alcohol, which has affected his mood and their business.

Maria told me that they do use mild physical punishment such as 'a slap if the children are naughty', but she believes that this has always been reasonable in the past. She told me that this was the first time Marius had 'ever hurt her children'. Stefan also told me that his father had 'never hurt him like this before'. The family have never had any contact with social care in the past.

Examination findings Stefan was dressed appropriately and appeared well kempt. He was quiet and obviously upset, but there appeared to be a comfortable rapport between Stefan and his mother. Maria was also tearful and very distressed by the situation. Stefan's weight was 37 kg (on the 50th centile) and his height was 147 cm (on the 75th centile). His pubertal staging was Tanner stage 2. On examination, four linear marks (0.3 cm × 5 cm), which had broken his skin, were seen lying obliquely on the front of his left thigh (labelled 1–4 on body map 1 (Figure 15.1). There was a large swelling on the front of his left thigh, consistent with a haematoma, which measured 6 cm × 5 cm (labelled 5 on body map 1 (Figure 15.1). There were six linear marks lying obliquely over his left forearm and hand, which had also broken his skin, each measuring 0.3 cm × 4 cm (labelled 6–11 on body map 2 (Figure 15.2), and a large dark swelling over his left upper arm, consistent with a haematoma, which measured 6 cm × 5 cm (labelled 12 on body map 2 (Figure 15.2). There were three linear marks over his back, each measuring 0.3 × 7 cm, which lay obliquely and had broken the skin (labelled 13–15 on body map 2 (Figure 15.2). No other abnormalities were seen on the remainder of the full examination.

Investigations X-rays of Stefan's left humerus and femur (upper arm and thigh) confirmed that there were no fractures. A full blood count and coagulation screen to see if Stefan had a bleeding problem were performed and were normal.

Overall impression and plan The findings seen on examination of Stefan Constantin were consistent with the history given of being whipped with an electric cable. The linear marks fit a history of being struck by the cable, and the two haematomas fit being struck by the plug. In my opinion considerable force was used to inflict these injuries.

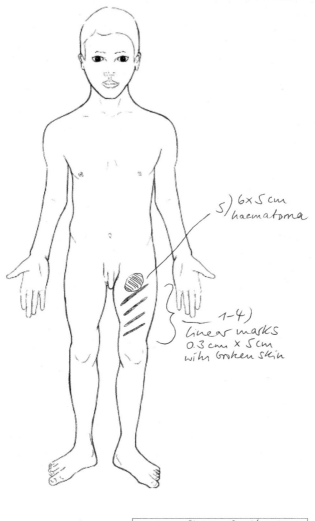

5) 6×5 cm haematoma

1-4) Linear marks 0.3 cm × 5 cm with broken skin

Patient name: Stefan Constantin

Date of birth: 4/3/2002

Date and Time of examination: 13/10/2014 9.30

Examining doctor: Katherine Fawbert

Examining Doctor's signature: KF.

Figure 15.1 Body map 1.

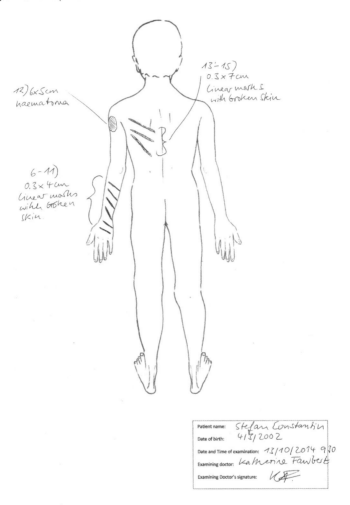

12) 6×5cm
haematoma

13-15)
0.3×7cm
Linear marks
with broken skin

6-11)
0.3×4cm
Linear marks
with broken
skin.

Patient name: Stefan Constantin
Date of birth: 4/8/2002
Date and Time of examination: 13/10/2014 9.10
Examining doctor: Katherine Fawbert
Examining Doctor's signature: KF

Figure 15.2: Body map 2.

Social care and the police need to complete their investigations. In my opinion Stefan, his sister Lacrimoara, and his mother Maria should be in a place of safety until investigations are complete. Stefan and his family may require psychological support, and I have given them sources of information. Their GP has also been informed with the consent of Maria, Stefan's mother.

Signed: Dr Katherine Fawbert.

Medical report writing resources

The RCPCH *Child Protection Companion* also gives an example medical report available online for members of the Royal College of Paediatrics and Child Health (RCPCH, 2013).

Conclusion

As a doctor involved in a case of potential child maltreatment your role is to carefully assimilate all the information gained in the history and examination of the child, together with any other sources of available information, such as any shared by social care. You are required to make a judgement, in discussion with other team members, about whether the examination findings fit plausibly with the history given. Overall, you need to decide if the picture fits consistently with a diagnosis of abuse *on the balance of probability*. Any decisions about next steps in dealing with the situation will be made as a team involving any relevant medical and social care professionals.

References

Children Act 1989 (c.41). London: HMSO.

Ministry of Justice. (2011). *Achieving Best Evidence in Criminal Proceedings: Guidance on Interviewing Victims and Witnesses, and Guidance on Using Special Measures*. London: Ministry of Justice.

RCPCH (Royal College of Paediatrics and Child Health). (2013). *Child Protection Companion* (2nd edn). Available at: http://www.rcpch.ac.uk/index.php?q=child-protection-companion (accessed 12 October 2014).

16

The safeguarding process: putting the jigsaw together

Ellie Day and Chloe Macaulay

Chapter summary

Once safeguarding concerns have been raised a process is initiated with the sole aim of ensuring that a child's well-being is preserved and they are protected from harm. This chapter will follow a child from when concerns are first raised through each step in the safeguarding process.

Case 16.1 First presentation

We first met Jasmine in Chapter 2 and are now going to follow her case (see Case 2.1 for the full presentation). Six-year-old Jasmine was brought to the Emergency Department by her mother, Rosemary, with recurrent abdominal pain. She was noted to be withdrawn and had a bruise on the rim of her ear. Her sister Isabel, nine years old, had a black eye. You raised child protection concerns.

> ### Case 16.1 Exercise
>
> ◆ Who is responsible overall for safeguarding these children?

Case 16.1 Discussion

Everyone has a responsibility for child safeguarding (see Box 16.1). Chapter 2 outlines the law regarding each individual's responsibility in this case. However, social care has the overall responsibility for determining the ongoing course of action.

Box 16.1 Safeguarding principles

♦ Safeguarding is everyone's responsibility; for services to be effective each professional and organization should play their full part.

♦ Safeguarding must have a child-centred approach; for services to be effective they should be based on a clear understanding of the needs and views of children.

As a medical professional, your priority must always be to ensure the immediate safety of the child/children. You are *not* responsible for deciding what happens next. All professionals must work together to assess children and follow the processes detailed in both government legislation and the policies of the local Safeguarding Children's Board.

Case 16.1 The next steps

You discuss Jasmine with Dr Sonali Gupta, the paediatric consultant on call. You then contact the out-of-hours duty social worker and explain your concerns about physical abuse and that you wish to make a referral. You provide the duty social worker with the names and dates of birth of all members of the family in order for background checks to be started.

An agreement is reached that Jasmine should be admitted overnight, but her siblings need a place of safety. The duty social worker discusses the case with the police Child Abuse Investigation Team and starts arranging a foster placement for Thomas and Isabel.

Case 16.1 Exercise

♦ What happens after a referral to social care has been made?

Case 16.1 Discussion

What happens after a referral to social care has been made?

Following the initial referral, social care has to decide whether there is sufficient evidence of significant harm to proceed. They base their assessment upon determining whether a referral meets the *threshold for concern* (see Box 16.2). They will often start with a *strategy meeting* to determine what is already known

---

Box 16.2

♦ Significant harm is the threshold that justifies compulsory intervention in family life in the best interests of children.

♦ Harm is defined as ill-treatment or the impairment of health or development.

---

and what the next steps should be. It is very important that health is part of that initial strategy meeting.

In many cases after a multi-agency discussion, it is felt that the situation does not meet the threshold and the escalation of child safeguarding procedures is halted. There is still a responsibility to assist and support the family, especially if areas of concern have been highlighted during the initial assessment. However, whenever there is reasonable cause to suspect that a child is at risk or is suffering significant harm, social care will start a formal process of assessment (Section 47 assessment).

Case 16.1 Further developments

Dr Sonali Gupta reviews Jasmine on the ward and shares your concerns. The duty social worker calls back and has some additional information regarding the family. The family is previously known to social care for domestic violence. The social worker is liaising with other local authorities to gather further information. The children's father, Matthew, has also been contacted. Thomas and Isabel, Jasmine's siblings, have been placed in foster care under police protection powers as the parents would not agree to a voluntary care agreement. Matthew is reported to be very angry, and the social worker advises that he is not permitted to visit the children. A strategy meeting is arranged for the next day. Rosemary is informed of the plan and is resident with Jasmine overnight. She is alarmed at the situation, and later a nurse hears her arguing with her husband on the phone.

Case 16.1 Exercise

♦ What are a police protection powers?

♦ What is a strategy meeting?

♦ What is an emergency protection order?

Case 16.1 Discussion

What are police protection powers?

When police officers have reasonable cause to believe that a child has suffered or could suffer significant harm, under Section 46 of the Children Act 1989 they may remove the child to suitable accommodation or take steps to prevent removal from a place of safety. Police powers to remove a child should only be used in exceptional circumstances relating to the immediate safety of the child and when there is insufficient time to seek an emergency protection order (see Table 16.1).

What is a strategy meeting?

A strategy meeting is a multi-agency planning meeting convened by social care. Social care will coordinate the meeting and other agencies, such as police, health, education, mental health, or probation, will be involved as necessary. The representatives from the police will usually be from the Police Child Protection Team, which is also known as Child Abuse Investigation Team. The agencies meet to share their concerns and gather any further information. Parents do not attend the meeting but it is best practice to inform them that it is taking place. A decision detailing what the next steps will be *must* be reached at the end of the meeting. The minutes are recorded on the Strategy Discussion Record and all agencies should receive a copy.

What is an emergency protection order?

If social care feels that it is necessary to remove a child from their home they must apply for an emergency protection order unless the delay would place the child at undue risk of harm (in which case police protection powers may be used). This is a court appointed order under Section 44 of the Children Act 1989. It is granted if the court is satisfied that there is reasonable cause to believe that a child is likely to suffer significant harm if they are not removed and placed in different accommodation, or if the child does not remain in their current 'safe' accommodation. Parental responsibility is given to the local authority, but at the same time it is not removed from the parents. Agencies must also consider the needs of the child (see Table 16.1).

Case 16.1 The strategy meeting and decisions

Following the referral, a social worker, Anwa Appadoo, is allocated and a strategy meeting is held on the ward the following day.

Table 16.1 Summary of orders used to safeguard children

Order	Definition	Time frame
Police protection powers	When there is immediate risk of harm or the child has suffered harm, under section 46 of the Children Act (1989), the police can remove a child to place of safety or take steps to keep a child in a place of safety.	Lasts 72 hours by which time, the local authority needs to apply for an emergency protection order or interim care order if the threshold for concern is met.
Emergency protection order	When a child is at risk of harm or has suffered harm, under Section 44 of the Children Act 1989, a local authority can apply to court for an emergency protection order allowing them to remove the child to a place of safety or keep them in a place of safety. This is a short-term measure.	Lasts eight days from the date of the court hearing and can be extended for a further seven days if the local authority reapplies to the court.
Child assessment order	Under Section 43 of the Children Act 1989, a child assessment order is available for local authorities to apply for when leading an investigation into the welfare, health, and development of a child. No court shall make a child assessment order if they are satisfied that there are reasonable grounds for making an emergency protection order. It is most commonly used when the child has suffered longer-term harm such as neglect rather than harm that is sudden and severe.	The maximum duration of a child assessment order is seven days from the date specified in the order with no power of extension.
Interim care order	A child can be placed with a suitable friend, a family member, or in care voluntarily under a Section 20 agreement (Children Act 1989). If the family refuses to agree to a voluntary placement, an interim care order (Section 31 of Children Act, 1989) can place the child in care on a temporary basis whilst the family is assessed and until the court can make a final decision about what is best for the child (see care order).	The Children and Families Act 2014 changed how long interim care orders lasted. Previously the order lasted for eight weeks and could be renewed every four weeks. The court can now specify how long the order lasts.

(continued)

Table 16.1 Summary of orders used to safeguard children (*continued*)

Order	Definition	Time frame
Care order	At the final hearing, the court must decide whether to make a full care order. To make a care order, the court must be convinced that the threshold criteria set out in Section 31 of the Children Act 1989 are met (i.e. that the child is suffering, or likely to suffer, significant harm and that the harm is attributable to the parents or carers). The court must also be convinced that making an order is better for the child than making no order at all—this is known as the 'presumption of no order'. A care order gives the local authority parental responsibility for a child.	Care orders last until: • the child's 18th birthday • an order is made giving parental responsibility to another person (e.g. through adoption) • the court lifts the order (this is called 'discharging' the order). Local authorities have a duty to continue to promote the welfare of care-leavers until the age of 21.
Supervision order	This order is made on the same basis as care orders but does not confer parental responsibility to the local authority. Under a supervision order it is the duty of the local authority appointed supervisor to befriend, advise, and assist the child, and to take steps to ensure that the child's needs are being met—for example, by ensuring that the child attends school and health appointments.	Initially lasts for one year, but the local authority can apply for renewal after one year up to a maximum of three years.
Adoption order	In circumstances where it would be unsafe for the child to return to live with her/his parents, the local authority may seek to have the child adopted. An adoption order (which transfers parental responsibility to the adoptive parents) is only made by a court following extensive enquiries. The sole criterion for deciding if the order should be made is the best interest of the child. At the point of the adoption the care order is discharged and the adoptive parents take over sole parental responsibility.	

The following professionals attend:

Social care	Anwa Appadoo: social worker
	Pierre Wright:children's services team manager
Health:	Sonali Gupta: paediatric consultant
	Clare Walton: ward sister
	Jane Westby: named nurse for safeguarding
	Georgina Holt: hospital liaison health visitor
Police:	DC Jude Hends: child abuse investigation team
School:	Jo Elsen: Jasmine's school nurse
Apologies	Dr Henry Haselgrove: GP

Pierre Wright chairs the meeting and asks Sonali Gupta to outline the reasons for Jasmine's admission and her concerns about physical abuse. Sonali Gupta reports that Jasmine's mother, Rosemary, said that Isabel had caused the marks on Jasmine's arm by pinching her. She offered no explanation for the bruise on Jasmine's ear. Jasmine was extremely withdrawn despite play specialist input. Isabel had a black eye which was not consistent with the explanation of being hit by Thomas with his beaker.

Anwa Appadoo, the allocated social worker, stated that the family is known following concerns raised by their neighbours who had reported a violent argument in the family's home six months ago. The family was also known to two neighbouring local authorities where they had previously lived, also for domestic violence.

Jo Elsen, the school nurse, said Rosemary had once rung Jasmine's school to authorize a friend to pick up the children because she was unwell. The following day she was seen with facial bruising, which she said occurred after she fell downstairs. Isabel's previous school had similar concerns about domestic abuse, but Rosemary had always denied that anything was wrong. In addition, Matthew, the children's father, had been intoxicated when picking them up from school more than once. She had notified their GP about her concerns.

Jude Hends, from the Child Abuse Investigation team, stated that Jasmine's father had a criminal record and had been to prison for assault. There were multiple reports of domestic violence, but these had been unsubstantiated and no charges had been brought. He was not known to have been violent towards the children.

Georgina Holt, the liaison health visitor, reported that all the children were up to date with their immunizations. Dr Henry Haselgrove sent a report that Rosemary had been seen for low mood and had been noted to have a black eye. He had suspected domestic abuse and had questioned her, but she had denied it. She had also failed to bring Jasmine for two speech therapy appointments.

Case 16.1 Exercise

- What concerns have been identified in the strategy meeting?

- What is a Section 47 enquiry?

- What is a Section 17 enquiry?

- What outcome options are available to the team in this case?

Case 16.1 Discussion

What concerns have been identified in the strategy meeting?

- Unexplained bruises and injuries

- A child of verbal age who is withdrawn and uncommunicative

- A history of alleged domestic abuse

- Family 'known' by number of local authorities

- Father has a criminal record for assault

- Father has history of alcohol intoxication

- Maternal low mood.

What is a Section 47 enquiry?

The purpose of the multi-agency strategy meeting is to decide whether the case meets the threshold for concern and therefore to escalate the process to a Section 47 enquiry (Section 47 of the Children Act 1989). It states that local authorities have a statutory responsibility to investigate whether action should be taken to safeguard or promote the welfare of a child.

Section 47 enquiries are conducted through a core assessment and carried out by an experienced child protection social worker. This builds on information already received and may require specific examinations by other professionals (medical, psychological, emotional, or developmental tests). Agencies such as health, police, and education have a responsibility to help and support in these enquiries. The outcome of a Section 47 enquiry may range from no further action, to further monitoring, to the convening of a child protection conference.

What is a Section 17 enquiry?

When there are lower-level concerns that a child is in need of early help and intervention but is not necessarily at risk of harm, social care may begin a Section 17 assessment. Section 17 of the Children Act 1989 stipulates that it is the general duty of every local authority to safeguard and promote the welfare of children in need. If a child is found to be disabled or the assessment finds that their health and development is likely to suffer without local authority intervention, the child will be classed as in need of support or intervention. A multidisciplinary assessment takes place led by social care who will speak to all those involved in the care of the children. It is considered a voluntary process (parental consent is needed to proceed). However, in practice, if parents refuse to comply with the process, it may be escalated to a Section 47 investigation.

What options are available to the team in this case?

1. **Section 47 enquiry and/or criminal investigation** If there is suggestion of criminal behaviour where an individual may be prosecuted, the strategy meeting may decide to start a criminal investigation. This will be led by the police with support and input from social care. This will run alongside a Section 47 enquiry as a dual-agency investigation.

2. **Section 17 enquiry** Children's services will proceed with a Section 17 investigation if there is reason to suspect that the children's needs are not currently being met or if they are unlikely to achieve or maintain a reasonable standard of health or development without intervention.

3. **No formal enquiry but assessment and provision of services.**

Case 16.1 Strategy meeting outcome

Pierre Wright, the Chair, hears everybody's views and concludes that there is enough evidence to proceed with a Section 47 enquiry. Everyone is in agreement. Child safeguarding medicals are booked for Isabel (see Chapter 17 for Isabel's safeguarding medical) and Thomas. Matthew, their father, is extremely angry about the outcome. He refuses to accept the findings. The children remain in foster care until the investigation is completed. A child protection case conference is set for 10 days time.

Case 16.1 Exercise

◆ What is a child protection case conference?

◆ Who can attend a case conference?

◆ What happens after a case conference?

Case 16.1 Discussion

What is a child protection case conference?

This is a multi-agency meeting convened typically as a part of the Section 47 enquiry. It should take place within 15 days of the strategy meeting.

It *aims* to bring together all the people who know the family to share information and talk about what is best for the child/children. It can also be convened before the birth of a baby deemed at potential risk or following significant concerns being raised regarding families already receiving support from services.

Its *purpose* is to ascertain if any changes are needed in order to ensure the safety and well-being of the child. It will strive to identify the strengths within the family and what actions the family themselves are able to deliver independently in order to achieve those necessary changes.

The meeting is led by a Chair who represents the Local Authority's Safeguarding Children's Board. The Chair is responsible for ensuring that all information is made available and everyone has an opportunity to contribute. Social care will present the background to the case along with a summary of the information collated and their analysis and recommendations. Every professional involved provides a report, which is particularly important for those who are unable to attend, and an opportunity to share it. The parents are also invited to contribute.

The *duty* of the conference is to decide upon an outcome. Every person involved will be invited to offer their opinion as to whether the child should be made subject to a child protection plan and, if so, which category/categories they will be placed under. Children can be placed under one or more categories of physical, emotional, neglect, or sexual abuse. It is rare to be placed under more than two categories.

Who can attend the child protection case conference?

Box 16.3 lists those who can attend a child protection case conference.

Box 16.3 Who can attend the case conference?

- The parents (with or without the child if appropriate)*
- Other family members*/a supporter*
- Social worker
- Police (if involved in a Section 47 enquiry)
- Family doctor (GP) and/or paediatrician
- Health visitor (or school nurse)
- Representatives from education (e.g. nursery staff, teacher, education welfare officer)
- Legal representatives (for the local authority or parents if required)
- Any other worker significantly involved with the family (e.g. probation officer, mental health worker)
- Interpreter (if required).

* As deemed acceptable by children's social services/the panel.

Case 16.1 The case conference

Jasmine's mother, Rosemary, attends the case conference. The children have all been living with a foster carer and she has had regular supervised visits. She has found it very hard to be separated from them. Following the strategy meeting, Mathew was physically abusive to her to such an extent that she required in-patient medical care. She states that she has finally realized that she herself is the victim of abuse and has agreed to press charges. He is currently on bail. She finally disclosed that the injuries found on Jasmine, including two healed cigarette burns, were caused by her husband. The police are conducting their own criminal investigation regarding the physical abuse. She has agreed to leave her husband and has signed a written agreement with social care. She agrees to the criteria set down by the case conference, and Jasmine, Isabel, and Thomas are returned to her care having been placed on a child protection plan for physical and emotional abuse.

Case 16.1 Exercise

- What happens after a case conference?

Case 16.1 Discussion

What happens after a case conference?

After the case conference, if it is felt that the child/children need to be subject to a formal child protection plan a *core group* will meet within 10 days of the conference to decide what services are required and how they will be provided. The group will include the parents, the social worker, and any other people from the key organizations who will be directly involved with the family.

This core group will meet regularly to ensure that services are being delivered and are addressing the needs raised at the conference. These meetings will continue regularly as long as the plan is in place.

A *review child protection conference* will meet within three months of the first conference to look at the progress made and determine whether the plan should continue or be altered. This review will be undertaken every six months until a decision is made that the child is no longer at continuing risk of harm.

If there are no further concerns about significant harm, the child comes 'off plan', and decisions are made about what other services they require. Once the child is removed from a child protection plan, the social worker will work with the family to determine what, if any, additional support services are required.

Conversely, if there are still significant concerns, the child protection plan should be revised and the process continues, with the core group being responsible for implementation of the plan. A further review conference should take place within six months. A child should not remain on a plan indefinitely as it is recognized that this is not in their best interests. If there is no change in the risk to the child/children over this period, social care may undertake legal planning for an interim care order (Section 31 of the Children Act 1989). If the local authority does choose to go to court, a children's guardian (an expert welfare officer) is appointed by the Children and Family Court Advisory and Support Service to look after the child's interests during the proceedings (see also Chapter 18).

Conclusion

The safeguarding process starts with a referral which can be made by anyone and is a multidisciplinary process led by social care. Everyone has a duty to play their part and, where possible, the parents should be actively encouraged to be involved. It is a complicated process involving significant inter-agency collaboration and communication, but clear guidance is available at both local and national level. Children's social care has overall responsibility for the process, but all agencies are duty bound to participate to ensure that the process runs efficiently and effectively. No individual agency or person has all the required knowledge to make an informed decision, but all the agencies involved by working together and communicating effectively will ensure that the child's best interests and welfare are maintained throughout.

References

Children Act 1989 (c.41). Available at: http://www.legislation.gov.uk/ukpga/1989/41/contents (accessed 8 August 2014).

Children and Families Act 2014. Available at: http://www.legislation.gov.uk/ukpga/2014/6/contents/enacted (accessed 26 November 2014.

HM Government (2013). *Working Together to Safeguard Children*. Available at: http//www.gov.uk/government/uploads/system/uploads/attachment_data/file/281368/Working_together_to_safeguard_children.pdf (accessed on 8 August 2014).

17

Medical record keeping

Gayle Hann

Note to reader

This chapter should be read with reference to Appendix 2 (Child protection medical assessment) and Appendix 6 (Body maps).

Chapter summary

This chapter outlines best practice in medical record keeping where there are child protection concerns. Following Royal College of Paediatrics and Child Health guidance (RCPCH, 2013), the use of a proforma (see Appendix 2) is recommended to standardize assessment and record keeping as well as to aid report writing. The importance of gaining consent for examination, medical photography, and information sharing will be covered. Included within medical record keeping is the practice of 'body-mapping', where injuries are recorded on a line drawing. This chapter will describe the best way to 'body map' a child so that injuries are clearly recorded and described for use in medical records, police statements, and court reports. Medical record keeping can also be improved by regular clinical governance activities such as the audit of patient notes.

Case 17.1 Medical record keeping in a case of physical abuse

In Chapter 2 we met Jasmine and her family. Jasmine was brought to the Emergency Department suffering from abdominal pain and safeguarding concerns were identified. At that time, her sister Isabel was noted to have a black eye. Anwa Appadoo, the allocated social worker, arranges a Section 47 medical for Isabel (see Chapters 15 and 16). You are the community paediatric registrar performing Isabel's medical. DC Jude Hends from the child abuse investigation team also accompanies Isabel and tells you that Isabel's mother is currently being interviewed. DC Hends asks you if she can have a copy of Isabel's notes and body map.

Case 17.1 Exercise

◆ How will you deal with consent for examination?

◆ What is the best way to document your consultation?

◆ How will you record Isabel's injuries?

◆ Are you allowed to give DC Hends a copy of Isabel's notes?

How will you deal with consent for examination?

Isabel's mother is currently being interviewed by the police, and it would be best to have written consent. You can ask the police officer to contact Isabel's mother so that you can gain consent over the telephone. Using the consent page of the medical proforma (see Appendix 2), you can ask Isabel's mother for consent in the presence of a witness, such as the social worker. You and the witness can then sign the consent page. This allows a full examination and documentation of findings which could not then be challenged later in court for reasons of inadequate consent.

What is the best way to document your consultation?

As soon as you have concerns that a child has suffered or is likely to suffer harm, the most effective way to record all your concerns is with a proforma (as outlined in Appendix 2). This example proforma conforms to the recommendations of the General Medical Council (GMC, 2013), the Royal College of Physicians (RCP, 2013), the Royal College of Paediatrics and Child Health (RCPCH, 2013), and many of the recommendations outlined in the Laming Report (2003) (see Table 17.1). Although example proformas, as outlined in Appendix 2 and RCPCH (2013), are lengthy, they meet all the information requirements needed in later social care referrals, police reports, and court reports (see Box 17.1).

Recommended documentation for any child where there are child protection concerns are:

◆ medical proforma (see Appendix 2)

◆ growth chart

◆ body maps (see Appendix 6)

◆ medical photography (if in hours and available).

Table 17.1 Good practice recommendations for medical record keeping

Recommendation
Clear contemporaneous notes should be made and if notes are being made by another person, the supervising doctor should review what has been recorded on their behalf.
Nursing care plans should document any child protection concerns.
Where the child is old enough to say what happened, the child should be talked to directly using open non-leading questions. Each question and response should be documented verbatim.
Where English is not the child's first language, an interpreter or a language line should be used.
Reasons for not talking to a child on their own or for not using an interpreter should be documented.
Any child that is admitted to hospital where there are child protection concerns should have a full and fully documented examination (including a 'body map') within 24 hours (unless doing so would compromise the child's physical or emotional well-being)
Admitting doctors should inquire about any previous hospital admissions or attendances where there are child protection concerns. If admissions or attendances have occurred at another hospital, those hospitals should be contacted for information about the attendance.
Where child protection concerns have been raised, assessment should not be considered complete until each concern has been addressed, accounted for, and fully documented.
All discussions about the child, including telephone conversations, should be kept in the child's notes (including discussions with social care, strategy meeting outcomes, discussions with parents or other carers).
If differences in opinion arise, discussions should be clearly documented and child protection concerns should not be rejected without full discussion, getting a second opinion if necessary.
If a child requires further investigations for child protection concerns, consent for those investigations should be sought by a doctor above the grade of a senior house officer.
Each child who is admitted for child protection concerns should have a named consultant who is clearly responsible for the child protection aspects of the child's care.
No child with child protection concerns should be discharged from hospital without discussion with their consultant or a paediatrician above the grade of a senior house officer.

(continued)

Table 17.1 Good practice recommendations for medical record keeping (*continued*)

Recommendation
All doctors involved in the care of a child with child protection concerns must provide social care with a written statement of the nature and extent of their concerns. If misunderstandings of medical diagnosis occur, these must be corrected in writing at the earliest opportunity.
Within a given location, health professionals should work from a single set of records for each child.
No child with child protection concerns should be discharged from hospital without a documented plan for their future care (see Appendix 7).
No child in which there are child protection concerns should be discharged from hospital without an identified GP.

Data from *The Laming Report of the Victoria Climbié Inquiry*, Recommendations 64–78, pp. 378–80
© Crown Copyright 2003.

How will you record Isabel's injuries?

On examination, Isabel's right eye is bruised and swollen shut. She has a small laceration within the swelling at the lateral edge of her right eyebrow. She also has a graze to her left knee and two small bruises on her right shin. She has a large bluish mark on her sacrum. The best way to document these marks is to draw and label them on a body map together with any explanation provided for how they happened (see Appendix 6 for blank sample body maps and also

---

Box 17.1 Golden rules for all medical record keeping

♦ Keep clear, accurate, and legible records

♦ Make notes at the time events happen or as soon as possible afterwards

♦ All documentation should have the relevant patient identifiers (name, date of birth, hospital, and NHS number) on both sides of each page

♦ Each entry should include the date, time, name of person documenting, their role, contact details, and signature

♦ Any mistakes should be crossed through with a single line, and signed and dated.

Isabel's body map (Figures 17.5 and 17.6). All marks/injuries should be measured with a tape measure.

In addition to the body map, describe the injuries in the section 'Abnormalities of the skin'. If you choose not to use a proforma, do use a body map and describe the marks and injuries found during your examination It is best practice to document your questions and answers verbatim in the notes.

Isabel's examination findings are described as follows:

Abnormalities of the skin

Abnormality 1 The right eye is swollen shut and is bruised. The lower lid is bluish-black in colour. The swelling itself measures 4 cm × 4.5 cm and extends onto the bridge of the nose. There is a 0.8 cm long by 0.1 cm wide laceration within the swelling on the outer edge of the eyebrow. An illustrated conversation between the doctor and Isabel about how her injuries occurred is shown in Figure 17.1.

Abnormality 2 There is a 2 cm × 3 cm graze to the left knee with brownish scabs on it. Figure 17.2 shows the conversation about this injury.

Abnormalities 3 and 4 There is a 1 cm × 1 cm brown bruise on Isabel's right shin, and a 1 cm × 2 cm brown bruise beneath injury 3 to Isabel's right shin. Figure 17.3 shows the conversations about these injuries.

Abnormality 5 There is a 4 cm × 6 cm bluish mark across the sacrum. Figure 17.4 shows the conversation about this injury.

The body maps (Figures 17.5 and 17.6) can be supplemented by medical photography. The police may choose to arrange their own photographer. The doctor should not take photographs on any personal device, such as a mobile phone, as this would breach the conditions of the consent as well as confidentiality.

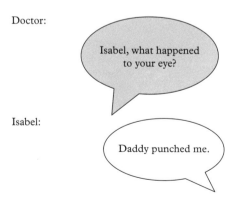

Figure 17.1 Explanation given for abnormality 1.

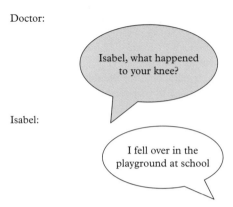

Figure 17.2 Explanation given for abnormality 2.

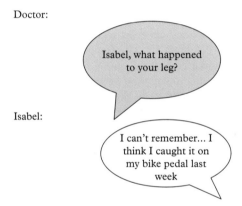

Figure 17.3 Explanation given for abnormalities 3 and 4.

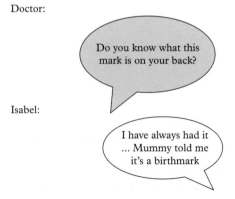

Figure 17.4 Explanation given for abnormality 5.

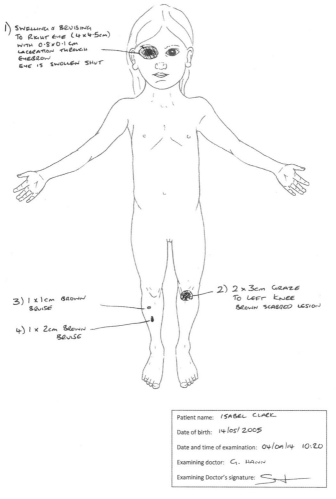

1) SWELLING & BRUISING
TO RIGHT EYE (4×4.5cm)
WITH 0.8×0.1 CM
LACERATION THROUGH
EYEBROW
EYE IS SWOLLEN SHUT

2) 2 × 3cm GRAZE
TO LEFT KNEE
BROWN SCABBED LESION

3) 1 × 1cm BROWN
BRUISE

4) 1 × 2cm BROWN
BRUISE

Patient name: ISABEL CLARK

Date of birth: 14/05/2005

Date and time of examination: 04/09/14   10:20

Examining doctor: G. HANN

Examining Doctor's signature: ⟨signature⟩

Figure 17.5 Body map 1.

Are you allowed to give DC Barton a copy of Isabel's notes?

Sharing information is essential in working to safeguard children. The doctor in this case should follow their hospital trust's protocol with regards to information sharing. If their trust does not have an information-sharing policy, this does not prevent the doctor from sharing information. Although doctors are

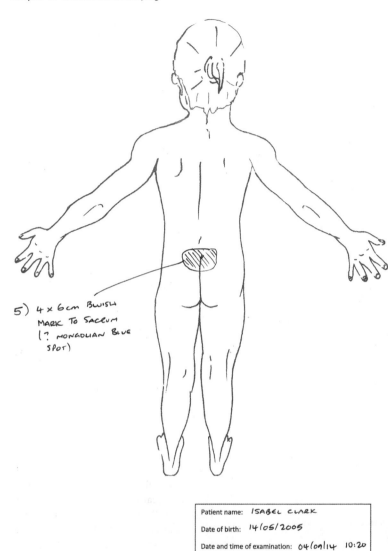

5) 4 x 6cm BLUISH MARK TO SACRUM (? MONGOLIAN BLUE SPOT)

Patient name: ISABEL CLARK

Date of birth: 14/05/2005

Date and time of examination: 04/09/14 10:20

Examining doctor: G. HANN

Examining Doctor's signature: _____

Figure 17.6 Body map 2.

bound by the principle of confidentiality, there is clear government guidance for frontline staff as to when information can be shared (DfE, 2008). Information can be shared without consent:

- if a child or adult is at risk of significant harm

- when a parent cannot care adequately or safely for a child

- if an individual is a risk to a child or adult

- when information shared, in addition to other information from a number of sources, allows agencies to come together and identify a child at risk.

Guidance published by the government (DfES, 2006), following the Laming Report of the Victoria Climbié Inquiry, stated that in general the law will not prevent you from sharing information with other practitioners if:

- those likely to be affected consent

- the public interest in safeguarding the child's welfare overrides the need to keep the information confidential

- disclosure is required under a court order or other legal obligation.

In this case, if you used the medical proforma contained in Appendix 2, two pages have been designed to be filled out as an interim report, together with the body maps, for the police and social worker to take away, as well as being an important part of the medical records.

Conclusion

The importance of clear, concise, and legible medical records cannot be stressed enough, particularly in the arena of child protection. This chapter provides clear guidance as well as the historical and legal background to child protection documentation. The Laming Report (2003) recommendations for documentation have been summarized, and should provide the minimum requirement for child protection documentation as well as providing audit standards. The use of a proforma is the best way to standardize your history, examination, and documentation of any child you see with child protection concerns. To summarize, if you haven't documented it, you haven't done it, and the evidence will simply not be there to be relied on in court.

References

DfE (Department for Education). (2008). *Information Sharing for Practitioners and Managers* Available at: http://webarchive.nationalarchives.gov.uk/20130401151715/https://www.education.gov.uk/publications/eOrderingDownload/00807–2008BKT-EN-March09.pdf (accessed 4 September 2014).

DfES (Department for Education and Skills). (2006). *What to Do If You Are Worried That a Child Is Being Abused*. Available at: https://www.gov.uk/government/uploads/system/uploads/attachment_data/file/190604/DFES-04320–2006-ChildAbuse.pdf (accessed 15 September 2014).

GMC (General Medical Council). (2013). *Good Medical Practice. Keeping Records*, paragraphs 52–60. Available at: http://www.gmc-uk.org/guidance/ethical_guidance/13427.asp (accessed 2 September 2014).

Laming. (2003). *The Victoria Climbie Inquiry: Report of an Inquiry by Lord Laming*. Available at: http://webarchive.nationalarchives.gov.uk/20130401151715/http://www.education.gov.uk/publications/eOrderingDownload/CM-5730PDF.pdf (accessed 3 September 2014).

RCP (Royal College of Physicians). (2013). *Standards for the Clinical Structure and Content of Patient Records*. Available at: https://www.rcplondon.ac.uk/sites/default/files/standards-for-the-clinical-structure-and-content-of-patient-records.pdf (accessed 2 September 2014).

RCPCH (Royal College of Paediatrics and Child Health). (2013). *The Child Protection Companion*. Available at: http://www.rcpch.ac.uk/child-protection-companion (accessed 31 January 2014).

18

Communicating concerns to parents

Ellie Day

Chapter summary

A positive partnership between parents and the safeguarding team is the fundamental principle underpinning the successful protection of children at every stage of the process. This chapter will focus on discussions with parents, including key strategies for preparation and helpful introductory sentences. It will help explain the child safeguarding procedure to the parents and provide information on the process to be understood from the family's perspective.

Breaking the news that there are safeguarding concerns is understandably something that doctors dread. The possible inflammatory nature of the discussion unnerves people, and if asked directly most people would probably say that they would defer it to another time or person if they possibly could. However, no one can or should avoid it. The assessment and discussion must be sensitive to the child's needs as well as those of the parents, and where appropriate the child must be informed about and feel able to participate in the process. In most instances it is good practice to involve the family from the start. Preparation and practice is key to getting it right (see Box 18.1 for strategies).

Case 18.1 Talking to parents

Holly is the four-month-old baby, whom we met in Chapter 14, Case 14.1, who was brought into the Emergency Department crying and not moving her right arm. An X-ray showed a spiral fracture of the humerus. The parents have no explanation for the injury.

You are the paediatric registrar who accepts the referral from the Foundation Year doctor, Amit Bhav, in the Emergency Department who had concerns as the parents were unable to explain how the injury had happened. Holly has been referred to the orthopaedic team and prescribed analgesia. When you fully

Box 18.1 Key strategies

Plan how you will broach the issues first

- Know what you want to say
- Be open and honest
- Provide clear explanations
- Remain confidential and professional
- Try to avoid jargon (child protection, safeguarding).

Plan how you might respond to the different reactions

- Anger
- Denial
- Emotional breakdown
- Fear.

Consider how your own anxiety will affect your communication

- Adapt your style to that of the parents:
  - ○ consider language barriers or learning difficulties.
- Consider the setting:
  - ○ Ensure that you introduce yourself clearly at the start
  - ○ Ascertain who is present in the room and their relationship to the child
  - ○ Consider the location for the discussion with emphasis on privacy, confidentiality, and safety (ensure that you position yourself nearest to the door or the panic button in potentially volatile situations).

undress her you find some bruises on her back. You have concerns that there is no mechanism to explain Holly's fractured humerus and make a referral to social care. The parents are asking when they can go home. Dr Bhav asks you if he can accompany you to talk to the parents to learn how to approach such a discussion.

Case 18.1 Exercise

- What words would you use to break the news that there are safeguarding concerns?

- How do you explain what will happen next?

Case 18.1 Discussion

What words would you use to break the news that there are safeguarding concerns?

You need to find the words and phrases that work for you, but you could say:

'Holly has broken her arm. The bone doctors will come and see her and we have given her some medicine for the pain. During the examination I have also found some bruises on her back. I am concerned by these injuries as I cannot fully explain how they were caused. We need to admit her to the ward as she needs more tests. Something we have to consider is whether this may have been caused by someone hurting her. I realize that this is difficult for you but we need your cooperation to get to the bottom of it. In these situations we often work with other teams to try and explore what might have happened, and this includes social care whom I have already contacted as part of the process. Nobody is accusing anyone, but for Holly's safety we have to ask you to work together with us.'

You have clearly explained what is wrong with Holly in a non-judgmental way without using medical jargon. Other possible opening sentences are outlined in Figure 18.1.

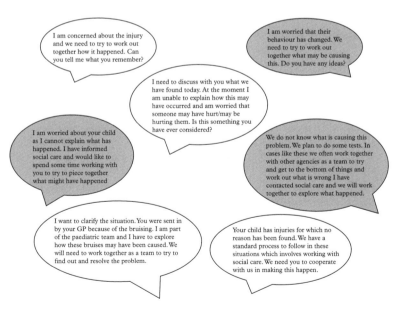

Figure 18.1 Useful phrases and words to communicate concerns to parents.

How do you explain what will happen next?

There are many ways of explaining what will happen next, but you could say:

'We have a clear protocol to follow in these situations. We have a legal and professional duty that we must uphold. I can provide you with information on this which may answer some of your questions. We would like you to help us with the process. This is a fact-finding mission that will contribute to an overall assessment which will help to guide us all and ensure that Holly is safe. We ask for your consent in proceeding forward. We need to do some investigations to look for any other injuries and see if there is any medical explanation for her injuries. I would like to explain what these entail. Do you have any questions?'

Case 18.1 Exercise

Holly's family have the following questions:

- What investigations will be done?

- When can we go home?

Case 18.1 Discussion

What investigations will be done?

Parents should consent to the examination and investigations. It is important to explain what the tests entail with a brief explanation of what can be expected in terms of the time frame for getting results, what the results will/won't tell you, and what will happen next. Examples of how you can explain what tests are needed are given in Figure 18.2.

When can we go home?

It is really important to explain the timeline to the parents once safeguarding concerns of any nature have been raised. Keeping them fully informed will help diffuse potential distress and distrust of the process. It will also help to manage their expectations on the approximate length of time that they can expect the process to take. Here is one example of how you could explain when they can take Holly home:

'I have spoken with children's social care and they are arranging an initial meeting for later today where we will discuss Holly's injuries. When Holly can go home will depend upon the results of the investigations. Social care will also

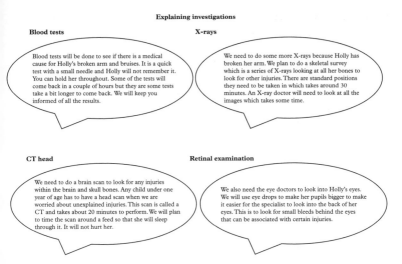

Explaining investigations

Blood tests

Blood tests will be done to see if there is a medical cause for Holly's broken arm and bruises. It is a quick test with a small needle and Holly will not remember it. You can hold her throughout. Some of the tests will come back in a couple of hours but they are some tests take a bit longer to come back. We will keep you informed of all the results.

X-rays

We need to do some more X-rays because Holly has broken her arm. We plan to do a skeletal survey which is a series of X-rays looking at all her bones to look for other injuries. There are standard positions they need to be taken in which takes around 30 minutes. An X-ray doctor will need to look at all the images which takes some time.

CT head

We need to do a brain scan to look for any injuries within the brain and skull bones. Any child under one year of age has to have a head scan when we are worried about unexplained injuries. This scan is called a CT and takes about 20 minutes to perform. We will plan to time the scan around a feed so that she will sleep through it. It will not hurt her.

Retinal examination

We also need the eye doctors to look into Holly's eyes. We will use eye drops to make her pupils bigger to make it easier for the specialist to look into the back of her eyes. This is to look for small bleeds behind the eyes that can be associated with certain injuries.

Figure 18.2 Useful phrases and words to explain the tests needed.

contact your GP and health visitor as part of the process before this meeting. After that it really depends upon what is decided at the meeting, but you will be kept fully informed. You will have an allocated social worker whom you will be able to contact and who can answer all your questions. They will also be able to provide you with contact details for some support and assistance for you during this process if you want it'.

Some parents will want to be informed about the legal framework for the assessment (see Chapter 16). Many local authorities have a detailed explanation of the procedures on their Local Safeguarding Children Board websites. Many have also produced information leaflets for parents.

Frequently asked questions

Will I lose my child?

This is the single biggest assumption that parents make when they are informed that there are child safeguarding concerns warranting investigation. However, in the majority of cases the children remain with the parents, and even those children subject to a child protection plan will remain in the family home. Children only need to be taken away from their home if information from a strategy meeting suggests there is an immediate danger and they cannot be protected within their own family.

It is the responsibility of the social worker to work with families to try and keep them together. However, if these measures fail, alternative options will be explored if the child is still perceived to be at risk. The first strategy employed is usually to explore whether there is a voluntary accommodation solution (Section 20, Children Act 1989) whereby it is agreed that the child will leave the family home and be looked after by someone else, usually a family member or friend, for a period of time.

If an agreement cannot be reached, social care will have to seek a court order in order to remove a child from the family home. Unless this is an emergency the family will usually be aware that a court order is being sought as they will receive a letter from the local authority before proceedings. This is a final notice for parents and is a means of encouraging them to work with social care to find a solution. In the majority of cases, even if a child is taken into care, social care will continue to work with the family so that the child can return home. A court order will dictate where a child should live and will also stipulate visitation rights and who can have contact with the child. Parents can appeal a care order directive but must do so within 21 days of its being announced.

What happens at court?

When a local authority makes an application for an order to safeguard the welfare of a child, the cases are usually referred to as public law cases and are initially heard in the Family Proceedings Court. This court is also responsible for awarding emergency protection orders. More complex cases may be transferred to a higher court, where decisions are made by judges. The court will appoint a children's guardian (an expert welfare officer) to look after the child's interests during the proceedings. The guardian is appointed by the Children and Family Court Advisory and Support Service (http://www.cafcass.gov.uk/about-cafcass.aspx) and is an independent person who is there to promote the child's welfare and ensure that decisions are in the child's best interests. If a child is judged to be sufficiently mature they will also be allowed to appoint a solicitor to represent their own wishes.

There are a number of different court orders that a local authority can apply for, but the most common are care orders, supervision orders, emergency protection orders, and secure accommodation orders (see Chapter 16, Table 16.1, for details and definitions of these orders).

What rights do parents have?

All parents have rights during the course of a child safeguarding enquiry. These include:

◆   to be treated with respect by professionals who have an open mind about relationships within the family

◆   to be given a clear explanation about what is happening and possible future action

- to have all decisions clearly explained

- to be listened to and to have their views asked for and recorded

- to be adequately supported by anyone they choose

- to seek legal advice

- to appropriate confidentiality

- to an appropriate interpreter if required

- to have their race, religion, and culture respected, taken into account, and carefully considered in any assessment

- to complain if they are not satisfied with the service they have received

- to see reports and assessments that social workers have written and have their views considered and noted.

Where can parents get help?

A lot of information is available online. Most local authorities and Local Safeguarding Children Boards have websites detailing their child protection procedures. A number of parent advice leaflets, detailing the process and including contact numbers and advice groups, are also available. The Ministry of Justice have a parents' pack entitled *Your child could be taken into care: Here's what you need to know,* which is available on the internet. Parents should be clearly directed towards these resources.

There are also organizations that are exclusively dedicated to helping parents going through care proceedings. These include the following:

- **The Family Rights Group** (http://www.frg.org.uk) is a charity that advises families who require social care input. They have a number of advice leaflets available and have also made some short films about the processes involved. They also offer an advice line which can be accessed.

- **Parentline Plus** (http://www.parentlineplus.org.uk) is a national charity that works for and with parents.

- **Coram Children's Legal Centre** (http://www.childrenslegalcentre. com) specializes in law and policy affecting children and young people. It is a national charity committed to promoting children's rights in the UK and worldwide. It has dedicated legal advice factsheets and call centres.

In addition there are a number of other organizations that can provide help and assistance to families. These include the following:

- NSPCC (http://www.nspcc.org.uk/help-and-advice/).

- Barnardo's.

- Samaritans.

Parents should be advised to seek legal advice at the start of any court proceedings if they have not done so before. If parents need legal advice there are a number of different agencies they can contact, including the following:

- A solicitor—there are many dedicated family law practices which specialize in child safeguarding procedures. Legal aid may be available (https://www.gov.uk/legal-aid/how-to-claim).

- Citizens Advice Bureau (http://citizensadvice.org.uk) provides a free website and face-to-face information and advice on legal, money, and other problems.

- Community Legal Advice (http://www.communitylegaladvice.org.uk).

- Family Justice Council (http://www.family-justice-council.org.uk).

- Coram Children's Legal Centre (http://www.childrenslegalcentre.com).

Conclusion

This chapter sets out techniques for communicating with parents, including useful words and phrases, when there are child protection concerns. Avoiding or delaying telling parents that you have concerns about abuse or neglect will increase the upset they will inevitably feel. Planned, open, and honest communication is best, using some of the techniques described in this chapter. However, the words and phrases suggested are just a helpful guide and you may find other phrases that work for you. A parent's greatest fear when social care becomes involved is that they will lose their child or children. As a health professional, it is essential that you familiarize yourself with the whole safeguarding process as well as where and who parents can turn to for support and advice. With this knowledge, you can continue to be their guide rather than their adversary, and it will reduce both your own and the parents' anxiety with the child protection process.

19

Appearing in court

Karen Aucott

Chapter summary

This chapter is an overview of appearing in court. It takes the reader through the whole process from receiving a request to give evidence to appearing as a witness. The chapter will explain the differences between courts, the difference between a witness of fact and an expert witness, the standards of proof required, the court process, and how to prepare for court, and will provide tips on giving evidence.

Introduction

If you are involved in child protection cases, you are likely to be called to court as a witness. The majority of people will attend as witnesses of fact, but some may appear as expert witnesses. A witness of fact will have been involved in the examination or treatment of the child and will be called upon to explain and expand upon their clinical opinion. Evidence will usually be based upon the medical report. A well written report will often prevent the need to appear in court. If you are called as a witness, it is usually because at least one person disagrees with something in your report. An expert witness will be called upon to provide an independent opinion on a case. They will base their report on a review of the case as well as a review of the published literature. Their opinion needs to be relevant (increases the likelihood that a particular fact is true or not) and needs to have sound scientific basis. The expert witness is paid for the work that they do and they must prove themselves credible in the face of the court. Trainees are often called as witnesses of fact, but do not have the knowledge or experience to be expert witnesses.

Case 19.1 Non-accidental head injury

One month ago you were the paediatric registrar on call when Joseph, a four-month-old boy, was brought into the paediatric emergency department. He was drowsy and floppy on arrival. His parents stated that he suddenly gave a high-pitched cry and then became floppy 'like a ragdoll' and had difficulty breathing. He had been snotty and taking fewer feeds over the previous 24 hours, but otherwise they had not noticed anything unusual. He had previously seen the health visitor because of concerns regarding reflux and not settling well.

After thorough examination and investigations, he was revealed to have multiple subdural haemorrhages on both acute CT and subsequent MRI scans of his brain. On ophthalmological examination, he had retinal haemorrhages. Medical differentials for these findings were excluded. After discussion with seniors, you concluded that the most likely diagnosis was non-accidental head injury and that the injury would fit with a shaking mechanism. You wrote a full medical report and a police statement.

Case 19.1 Request to appear in court

You have now received a letter from the county court asking you to give evidence. The local authority's instructing solicitor has requested that a copy of the notes and all imaging is provided to the court.

Case 19.1 Exercise

♦   What should you do to prepare yourself for court?

Case 19.1 Discussion

What should you do to prepare yourself for court?

♦ Obtain the original notes and your medical report and familiarize yourself with the case.

♦ Check that the report is factually correct compared with the written notes. If there are any discrepancies, it is important to send an addendum to your report addressing the matter; this may also include whether any difference of opinion has been raised following peer review.

♦ Contact the Trust's named doctor to discuss the case.

♦ You can also contact your medical defence union to check your report (this is a useful and often under-utilized service).

♦ In a criminal case:
   ○ you can ask the police for a copy of your statement if you did not take a copy
   ○ if you are appearing for the prosecution, you can contact the Crown Prosecution Service for advice and a copy of your statement.

Case 19.1 Seeking advice on appearing in court

You contact the named doctor for child protection; a colleague has told you that as this case is being heard in a county court, it is a more serious case. You ask the named doctor to explain the differences between the courts.

Case 19.1 Exercise

- What are the differences between the courts and their function?

- What should you wear to court?

- Who will be there and what will happen?

- What happens if your evidence isn't strong enough to support the local authority?

- Any tips for giving evidence?

Case 19.1 Discussion

What are the differences between the courts and their function?

The named doctor explains that as this case is being heard in county court, the instructing solicitor is employed by the local authority. This is a civil case where the local authority are seeking to obtain a care order for Joseph. A criminal case may be brought later in the magistrates' court for which you may also be called to give evidence.

The court system is divided into criminal courts and civil courts. Criminal courts decide whether a defendant is guilty of committing a crime, and civil courts resolve issues regarding private matters between individual people or organizations. Family courts are a subsection of the civil courts. Their role is to resolve disputes between two parties, for example the local authority and a parent, or in private law between parents. Civil cases are generally heard in the county court and will be decided by a district or circuit judge.

Criminal cases are generally heard in a magistrates' court and will be decided by a district judge or magistrates. Magistrates may be legally qualified or lay people who volunteer their services and do not require formal legal qualifications. They are given legal advice by qualified clerks (Judiciary, 2014a). More serious criminal cases are passed on to the Crown Court and are decided by a judge and jury. The judge decides matters regarding the law and the jury decides matters of fact.

Most child protection cases will be public law cases brought by local authorities, as in Joseph's case, and include matters based on safeguarding or promoting the welfare of children. The aim of the hearing is to identify whether a significant threshold has been met in order for the local authority to intervene to safeguard the child or to decide on the best care plan for that child (care order, supervision order, or emergency protection order). Public law cases must start in the family proceedings court but may be transferred to the county court if it will minimize delay, if there is disputed expert evidence, or where the case is exceptionally complex (Judiciary, 2014b).

The burden of proof rests with the prosecution (the local authority in civil courts and the Crown Prosecution Service in criminal courts). The prosecution must prove their case and the defence must answer to it. In *civil courts* the burden of proof is based on the *balance of probability* (i.e. it is more likely than not that the injury was acquired non-accidentally). In *criminal courts* the burden of proof must be *beyond all reasonable doubt* and therefore the evidence needs to be much stronger.

What should you wear to court?

You should look professional when attending court and should dress as you would for a professional interview. A plain dark suit is recommended by the Bond Solon legal training company, who provide courses for both witnesses of fact and expert witnesses.

Who will be there and what will happen?

In all family courts:

- solicitor/barrister for each party

- local authority legal advisor (solicitor)

- children's guardian

- witnesses of fact

- expert witnesses.

You will initially be asked to take an oath (religious) or an affirmation (non-religious) in which you swear to tell the truth. You will be asked questions by the prosecution initially and these will be followed by a cross-examination by the defence. A summary will be made by the prosecution and further questions may be asked at this time.

What happens if my evidence isn't strong enough to support the local authority?

You do not need to worry about letting anyone down. You are there to provide independent evidence to the courts to assist them in making a judgement on the case; you are not there to represent one particular party or to give an opinion as to what you think should happen or what the outcome should be.

Any tips for giving evidence?

Know your report well and familiarize yourself with any evidence on the subject matter. Listen carefully to the questions and ask for clarification if you don't understand. Face the judge and present your answers to him/her. Tell your story remembering that you are there to give evidence, and are not on trial. Be patient during cross-examination and do not become defensive. Your testimony should be fair and balanced.

Case 19.1 The day of the court case

On the day of the court case, you arrive early. Despite your preparation, you do not know where to go or when you will be required to give evidence.

Case 19.1 Exercise

◆ What help is available to you?

◆ How will you know when to give evidence?

◆ How should you address the judge?

Case 19.1 Discussion

What help is available to you?

A list will be available within the courts detailing which courtroom each case is being heard in. You should report to the usher at the relevant courtroom. Any questions about the court process can be directed towards the usher or the legal advisor.

How will you know when to give evidence?

You will be called and directed to the witness stand.

How should you address the judge?

Ask the usher to let you know before you are sworn in, but typically:

♦ magistrates/district judge   Sir/Madam

♦ circuit judge   Your Honour.

Case 19.1 Giving evidence

You are asked to summarize your involvement with the case, and then are asked the following questions by the prosecution (Appendix 3 contains the actual court report).

Can a mechanism for identifying the injuries be identified?

As a registrar, you will not be expected to know all the evidence on non-accidental head injuries but it is fair for you to state that, based on your experience and background reading, shaking episodes in young children often show characteristic findings of subdural haemorrhages (bleeds around the brain) in combination with retinal haemorrhages (bleeds to the back of the eye), as were found in this case. Despite extensive investigation, no alternative explanation has been found to account for the injuries and you believe that the most likely mechanism is shaking.

Could the injuries have occurred without any physical signs being apparent to the caregiver?

You may not be able to answer this question fully as you are a witness of fact. However, if you feel comfortable, you may state that a child who has been shaken with sufficient force to cause subdural haemorrhages and retinal haemorrhages is likely to have shown some physical signs (as well as being distressed at the time of the incident) but, depending on the size of the bleed, these signs may have been subtle, such as lethargy and poor feeding. If you do not feel comfortable stating an opinion, you should say so. An expert witness may be able to answer this more fully.

Subsequently, you are called to give evidence at the criminal court as the parents are to be prosecuted. You are asked the following questions by the prosecution.

Is it possible to identify the date each injury was caused?

Again, you may feel comfortable answering this question, but you should be careful not to go beyond your level of knowledge or expertise. You may state that as Joseph presented acutely with an episode of a high-pitched cry, followed by a sudden silence, subsequent floppiness, and laboured breathing, it is likely that a shaking injury occurred shortly before this episode. The subsequent floppiness and laboured breathing are likely to be a consequence of the bleed into the head. An expert opinion may be sought from a neuroradiologist on the findings of the CT and MRI scans.

Assuming that the injury was caused by shaking, can you articulate the severity of the shaking or the length of time the shaking lasted?

This question is likely to require an expert witness to answer. You may state that, based on your previous experience and reading, considerable force would be needed whilst shaking a baby to cause subdural haemorrhages and retinal haemorrhages—these are not findings that are found as a result of routine care or playful bouncing or jumping around with a baby.

Could earlier medical treatment have resulted in less permanent damage to the child?

As a registrar, you should again be careful not to exceed your knowledge and level of experience. You may state that at the current time it is difficult to pre-dict the child's long-term prognosis or whether earlier intervention would have resulted in a different prognosis.

Comment on your evidence

Your evidence would have been better presented if you could have backed it up with some evidence-based medicine. This would have supported your clinical reasoning and the preparation would have improved your credibility as a wit-ness. Have a look at the example court report in Appendix 3 based on the same case study. This gives more detailed answers and may have avoided the need for oral evidence.

In the criminal court, you may also have been asked further questions on the detail of the CT scan (time frame, location of haemorrhages, and relation to injury) or on the degree of force needed and any evidence base. It is important that you do not try to answer questions that are beyond your level of knowledge/ expertise or use an evidence base that you are not familiar with to support your answers. These are questions that you should refer to an expert witness or a col-league with more expertise in that area.

Note that in civil courts questions are likely to be based around whether it is likely that the care given to the child has been below the standard expected and whether there is enough evidence to support the local authority intervening (causation of injuries, elimination of alternative diagnoses, appropriate response from caregivers). In criminal courts, questions are more likely to be asked to elicit whether the injuries can be attributed to a specific person/s (i.e. elim-ination of alternative diagnoses), the timing (important for opportunity to harm), and the impact on the child and the prognosis (sentencing, compensation).

Further information on courses available can be found in Chapter 20 on child protection training. The Royal College of Paediatrics and Child Health runs a two-day face-to-face course in conjunction with the legal training company Bond Solon.

Conclusion

Many healthcare professionals dread being asked to give evidence in court. However, if you follow the guidance given in this chapter and write a clear and concise witness statement, your appearance may not even be required. If you are subsequently asked to appear in court, you will find yourself guided through your statement in a systematic fashion by the barrister leading the prosecution. Cross-examination is often feared, but usually occurs to establish a timeline or who caused the injury. It is important to stay within the facts of your written statement without straying outside your knowledge base. You may state your opinion whether you are a professional or an expert witness, but you can be asked to qualify your opinion. There is no shame in stating that you simply do not know the answer or that the answer lies beyond your expertise. Expert witnesses must also stay within the boundaries of their knowledge, although this knowledge is more extensive.

References

Judiciary (2014a). *Magistrates' courts*. Available at: http://www.judiciary.gov.uk/you-and-the-judiciary/going-to-court/magistrates-court (accessed 8 April 2014).

Judiciary. (2014b). *Family courts*. Available at:http://www.judiciary.gov.uk/you-and-the-judiciary/going-to-court/family-law-courts (accessed 8 April 2014).

20

Child protection training

Arabella Simpkin and Gayle Hann

Chapter summary

All staff who come into contact with children and young people have a responsibility to safeguard and promote their welfare and to know how to act on any concern (RCPCH, 2014). This underlying principle pivots around sharing concerns on a multi-agency basis, developing solutions, and maintaining safety networks for children and their families.

Introduction

Why have child protection training?

♦ To ensure that safeguarding concerns are recognized and acted upon in line with best current practice.

♦ To ensure that health professionals have adequate training and support, as this has been cited as a reason for ongoing concerns (GMC, 2012).

♦ to gain access to peer review, clinical supervision, and emotional support so that health professionals are confident and competent in this stressful and demanding area of work.

♦ Child protection continues to evolve with changes in knowledge and practice; hence there is a need for regular updates and further training to ensure that health professionals have adequate knowledge of the resources available.

What training is needed for different levels?

Safeguarding competences are the set of abilities that enable professionals to effectively safeguard, protect, and promote the welfare of children and young people. Acquiring knowledge, skills, and expertise in safeguarding/child protection should be seen as a continuum.

Box 20.1 Competency Framework

Level 1 All staff working in healthcare settings

Level 2 All non-clinical and clinical staff who have any contact with children, young people, and/or parents/carers

Level 3 All clinical staff working with children, young people, and/or their parents/carers and who could potentially contribute to assessing, planning, intervening, and evaluating the needs of a child or young person and parenting capacity where there are safeguarding/child protection concerns

Level 4 Specialist roles—named professionals

Level 5 Specialist roles—designated professional groups

Level 6 Board Level for chief executive officers, Trust and Health Board executive and non-executive directors/members, commissioning body directors

A full copy of the document can be found in RCPCH (2014).

Reproduced from Royal College of Paediatrics and Child Health, *Safeguarding Children and Young People: Roles and Competences for Health Care Staff*, p. 10 © Royal College of Paediatrics and Child Health, 2014.

Six levels of competence are described by the framework devised by the Royal College of Paediatrics and Child Health (RCPCH, 2014) (see Box 20.1). The competencies are gained in a stepwise fashion—thus those requiring skills at level 5 will also have gained competency at levels 1 to 4. Please refer to the full guidance if you are unsure about what level of training you should have.

Case 20.1 Level 1: Non-clinical staff working in a healthcare setting

Stephanie is working as the receptionist in the adult outpatient clinic when she witnesses a father slapping his three-year-old son, Jake. Stephanie is concerned by the force and anger with which the father addresses the child and at the end of the clinic she phones you for advice. You are the paediatric registrar on call.

Case 20.1 Exercise

- What should you advise Stephanie to do?

- What training is available for her?

Case 20.1 Discussion

What should you advise Stephanie to do?

Stephanie undoubtedly has a duty to report this incident and share her concerns. The person who should make a referral should be the person who holds the most information about the child, and that person is Stephanie as she witnessed the incident. However, as an ST4 (Specialty Trainee Year 4), you have more experience than Stephanie and so you could guide her through the process.

What training is available for her?

◆ A mandatory session of at least 30 minutes duration should be included in every general staff induction programme, highlighting who to contact and seek advice from in the event of any concerns. Everyone should receive a minimum of 2 hours refresher training every three years.

◆ Introduction to safeguarding children and young people:

○ Interactive session of about 30 minutes

○ Online—delivered by e-Learning for Healthcare in partnership with the RCPCH (http://www.e-lfh.org.uk/projects/safeguarding-children)

○ Free of charge for NHS employees.

Case 20.2 Level 2: ST1 paediatric trainee

You are an ST1 paediatric trainee who sees two-year-old Abdul in the paediatric emergency department with a burn to the right thigh. The mother is unsure how the burn occurred, but thinks it may have been from a hot water bottle that leaked three days ago. It is superficial and requires dressing and analgesia. Because of the delay in presentation and lack of clarity as to the mechanism of injury, you discuss the case with your registrar who advises you to make a social care referral. You are unsure how to tell his mother, as you are worried that she will think that you are accusing her of non-accidental injury.

Case 20.2 Exercise

◆ What can you do to help increase your confidence?

◆ What courses exist to give you the skills to recognize and act on child protection concerns?

Case 20.2 Discussion

What can you do to help increase your confidence?

The Child Protection Recognition and Response course, run by the Advanced Life Support Group (ALSG), offers the opportunity for face-to-face practice scenarios in a non-intimidating environment with feedback from senior paediatricians. Role-playing activities and small-group workshops provide a forum for gaining confidence in this challenging area. A mentor system which allows any queries to be answered throughout the day is available.

What courses exist to give you the skills to recognize and initiate child protection concerns?

◆ **Recognition, Response, and Record**

  ○ Consists of three 30-minute e-learning sessions

  ○ Online—delivered by e-Learning for Healthcare in partnership with the RCPCH (http://www.e-lfh.org.uk/projects/safeguarding-children)

  ○ Free of charge for NHS employees.

◆ **Child Protection, Recognition, and Response**

  ○ Three topics to be studied online followed by a pre-course multiple choice question (MCQ) test prior to the face-to-face course

  ○ One-day face-to-face course: lectures, workshops, role plays, scenarios, structured approach to child protection cases

  ○ Apply for course on the ALSG website (http://www.alsg.org).

Case 20.3 Level 3: Paediatric registrar

You are a paediatric registrar performing a child protection medical for 13-year-old Veronica, who has made allegations that her mother hits and punches her. Veronica has been placed in emergency foster care. On clinical examination you notice that there are several scratch marks over Veronica's arms and face, and she has bruises on her stomach. You are asked to attend a strategy meeting and are worried as you have never had the opportunity to attend a strategy meeting or case conference and are unsure what will be expected of you.

Case 20.3 Exercise

◆ What will be expected of you at the strategy meeting?

◆ What training is available for your level?

Case 20.3 Discussion

What will be expected of you at the strategy meeting?

Chapter 16 describes in detail what happens at strategy meetings as well as the subsequent outcomes. You should ensure that you have all the relevant information regarding Veronica with you at the meeting. The aim of the meeting will be to put together a plan on whether a core assessment under Section 47 of the Children Act 1989 should be carried out. You will be asked to summarize your findings from the clinical examination and state your opinion as to whether Veronica is a victim of physical abuse.

If you have not attended a strategy or professionals meeting before, it is best to take someone with you who has. Usually the named doctor or nurse for child protection will be willing to support you. You will receive a copy of the minutes after the meeting and you should check that they record your concerns accurately.

What training is available for your level?

◆ **Maintaining and Updating Competencies**
  ○ Seven e-learning sessions covering a wide range of topics delivered by e-Learning for Healthcare in partnership with the RCPCH (http://www.e-lfh.org.uk/projects/safeguarding-children)
  ○ Free of charge for NHS employees.

◆ **Child Protection in Practice**
  ○ Nationally recognized two-year online educational programme for speciality trainees
  ○ Programme modules (each can take up to four months to complete)
  ○ Each module can be bought individually
  ○ Apply for the course on the ALSG website (http://www.alsg.org).

◆ **Child Protection: From Examination to Court**

○ Two-day face-to-face course at the RCPCH designed for senior trainees (ST6+)

○ Book a place at http://www.rcpch.ac.uk/events/child-protection-examination-court.

◆ **Evening of Evidence Series**

○ Delivered by RCPCH

○ Book online at http://www.rcpch.ac.uk/events-courses/rcpch-events-courses/evenings-evidence-series/evenings-evidence-series.

Case 20.4 Levels 4 and 5: Named professional

We revisit the case of Holly from Chapter 14.4, Case 14.1, and Chapter 18, Case 18.1. Holly is a four-month-old baby who has been admitted for investigation of a spiral fracture of the humerus. The only mechanism of injury provided was an episode of crying after being strapped into her car seat a few days earlier, an event that she had settled quickly from. Examination had revealed two circular bruises on her right arm and a few small bruises on her back. The paediatric consultant, Dr Jones, is overseeing the rest of her admission and investigations.

Case 20.4 Exercise

You are the named doctor for child protection and your colleague Dr Jones has asked your advice about the injury as she is writing a report for social services and will be attending a case conference. She is unsure of how indicative of abuse a humeral fracture is.

◆ Where can you go for information to guide your colleague on the likelihood that the fracture is abusive?

◆ What are the expectations of you in your role as named professional?

Case 20.4 Discussion

Where can you go for information to guide your colleague on the likelihood that the fracture is abusive?

The Cardiff CORE INFO website (http://www.core-info.cardiff.ac.uk/), which you have previously used as a resource to review the literature, agrees with the guidance and states that spiral fractures in the humerus in children aged less than five years are strongly associated with abuse. As described in Chapter 14, Case 14.1, a systematic review demonstrated that the risk of a humeral fracture being abusive in a child less than three years was one in two, and a spiral fracture was the most common abusive fracture of the humerus in a child under 15 months of age (Kemp et al., 2008).

You now feel that you have the evidence-based information needed to guide your colleague (see Box 20.2).

What are the expectations of you in your role as named professional?

◆ To participate regularly in support groups or peer support networks for specialist professionals at a local and national level.

◆ To complete a management programme with a focus on leadership and change management within three years of taking up your post.

◆ In addition to training programmes, you should circulate written update briefings and literature as appropriate to all staff at least annually.

Box 20.2 Resources to guide evidence-based practice

◆ **Cardiff Child Protection Systematic Review** (http://www.core-info. cardiff.ac.uk):a series of systematic literature reviews of physical abuse and neglect in children.

◆ **British Association for the Study and Prevention of Child Abuse and Neglect** (BASPCAN) (http://www.baspcan.org.uk).

◆ **National Society for the Prevention of Cruelty to Children** (NSPCC) (http://www.nspcc.org.uk/core-info):a series of leaflets based on the Cardiff Child Protection Systematic Review.

◆ **Current Awareness Service for Policy, Practice and Research** (CASPAR) is run through the NSPCC website and gives the latest news regarding developments in child protection—you can sign up for email alerts.

◆ **Child Abuse Professional Network** (CAPnet).

◆ **General Medical Council** (GMC) consultation on new child protection guidance: *Protecting Children and Young People: The Responsibilities of all Doctors* (GMC, 2012).

◆ **National Institute for Health and Clinical Excellence (NICE)** guideline CG89 *When to Suspect Child Maltreatment* (NICE, 2009): this gives both a summary of how to recognize child abuse and reviews the evidence.

Level 6

Experts should undertake specific training on the role of the expert witness in the courts.

Where can this training be achieved?

◆ Training can be obtained from professional organizations (e.g. the Royal College of Psychiatrists and RCPCH) or accredited independent providers.

◆ Expert witnesses in child protection

  ○ Two-day face-to-face course at the RCPCH (Child Protection: From Examination to Court)

  ○ Aimed at experienced paediatricians who have previously appeared as expert witnesses or have aspirations to do so.

Additional training (relevant for all levels)

◆ National Learning Management System (NLMS):an e-learning platform centrally funded by the Department of Health and free of charge

◆ Local health organizations run safeguarding children training programmes

◆ National courses:

  ○ Child Protection Special Interest Group (CPSIG)—http://www.cpsig. org.uk

  ○ National Society for the Prevention of Cruelty to Children (NSPCC)—http://www.nspcc.org.uk

  ○ British Association for the Study and Prevention of Child Abuse and Neglect (BASPCAN)— http://www.baspcan.org.uk.

◆ MSc modules in child health

◆ Multi-agency Local Safeguarding Children Board (LSCB) training

◆ Healthsafeguarding.com organize courses for all levels including named and designated doctors

◆ Safeguarding Children e-Academy—http://www.safeguardingchildrenea.co.uk

◆ Training with the judiciary for a better understanding of court process and help to prepare for future court hearings

◆ Rosie 1 and 2: child protection simulation 'games' developed by the University of Kent Centre for Child Protection which offers a new interactive way for professionals to evaluate child protection situations—http://www.kent.ac.uk/sspssr/ccp/game/rosie1index.html.

Conclusion

There is clear guidance from the RCPCH on the knowledge and training that each health professional requires in safeguarding and child protection. Every hospital is required to train their staff in child protection according to these competencies, as well as publishing their figures on their Trust's dashboard. However, despite these institutional requirements, it is your personal responsibility to ensure that you have adequate training in order to identify and respond to child abuse. This chapter has summarized the different levels of knowledge required by all health professionals who work with children. A wide variety of training courses and resources are available, both online and face to face, to cater for different learning styles. Whatever level of training you require, you must keep up to date with changes in both child protection policy and the law in order to both revalidate and keep children safe.

References

GMC (General Medical Council). (2012) *Protecting Children and Young People: The Responsibilities of All Doctors*. Available at: http://www.gmc-uk.org/guidance/ethical_guidance/13260.asp (accessed 14 July 2015).

Kemp, A.M., Dunstan, F., Harrison, S., et al. (2008). Patterns of skeletal fractures in child abuse: systematic review. *British Medical Journal*, **337**, a1518.

NICE (National Institute of Clinical Excellence). (2009). *When to Suspect Child Maltreatment*. Available at: http://www.nice.org.uk/CG89 (accessed 31 October 2014).

RCPCH (Royal College of Paediatrics and Child Health). (2014). *Safeguarding Children and Young People, Roles and Competences for Health Care Staff*. Available at: http://www.rcpch.ac.uk/system/files/protected/page/Safeguarding%20Children%20-%20Roles%20and%20Competences%20for%20Healthcare%20Staff%20%2002%200%20%20%20(3)_1.pdf (accessed 31 October 2014).

21

Child protection: when things go wrong— serious case reviews

Eleanor Perera

Chapter summary

This chapter will cover the process of a serious case review. It will give practical advice for professionals, illustrated by the lessons learned from a high profile-case (Daniel Pelka, 2012), and present common themes emerging from other serious case reviews.

Please note that the case described is real and the information discussed is published and freely available to the general public. The authors gratefully acknowledge the transparency of the agencies involved in facilitating others to learn from this case, which reflects their 'strong commitment to work towards improving practice in the future' (Wonnacott, 2014).

Case 21.1 Daniel Pelka

Daniel died on 3 March 2012, aged four years and eight months. His mother and stepfather, who set out to deliberately harm him and lie to professionals, were found guilty of his murder. Their callousness and deception was reflected in the sentencing, with each receiving a minimum term of 30 years (*R v Krezolek and Luczak*, 2013). Pathological examinations revealed an acute subdural haematoma, an older subdural haemorrhage, 40 injuries in total, gross malnourishment, and dehydration. He had been subjected to neglect and abuse for a prolonged time. The family had been known to a number of agencies, and subsequently a serious case review was carried out. However, details of the systematic abuse that he underwent only emerged at the criminal trial.

Case 21.1 Exercise

♦ What is a serious case review?

♦ Who conducts the review?

♦ Who can see the findings?

♦ What are the criticisms of serious case reviews?

Case 21.1 Discussion

What is a serious case review?

Local Safeguarding Children Boards (LSCBs) in England are statutorily required to carry out a serious case review when a child has died or been seriously harmed and abuse or neglect is suspected to be involved, and there is concern about how agencies worked together in safeguarding the child (HM Government, 2006). The key purpose is to ensure that lessons are learned; it is neither a public enquiry nor a disciplinary process. The professionals and organizations involved with the child should be engaged in the process, without fear, and families invited to contribute (HM Government, 2015). Biennial analyses of serious case reviews in England are available from the Department for Education.

Who conducts the review?

The serious case review is led by one (or more) qualified independent individuals who analyse individual management reviews conducted by each agency involved. The exact methodology for conducting the review is determined by the LSCB, but they should aim for completion within six months of its initiation (HM Government, 2015). The methodology for conducting individual management reviews, detailed in *Working Together* (HM Government, 2010), relies on access to the records, highlighting the importance of documentation.

Who can see the findings?

Working Together (HM Government, 2015) advises that all serious case review reports should provide sound analysis, must be published in plain English, and must be freely available. The LSCB should monitor and report the implementation of actions by agencies.

What are the criticisms of serious case reviews?

Criticisms (Brandon et al., 2011) have suggested that recommendations

- are numerous

- pertain only to individual cases

- are not evidence based

- are prescriptive in nature, seldom tackling the complexities of professional judgement.

Working Together (HM Government, 2010) advised that recommendations should be few, focused, and specific. The Munro Review (Munro, 2011) recommended that serious case reviews should be conducted using a systems-based methodology to determine not only what went wrong, but why the system allowed it.

Case 21.1 Daniel Pelka: the serious case review

Case 21.1 Exercise

In this exercise we shall examine the serious case review conducted following Daniel's death (Lock, 2013), answering the questions:

- What were the key findings?

- What can paediatricians learn from this serious case review?

- What were some of the key recommendations?

Case 21.1 Discussion:

What where the key findings?

The serious case review process was finalized prior to the criminal trial and additional information was incorporated into the report. A further deeper analysis (Wonnacott, 2014) was completed following the publication of the serious case review.

Professionals Practitioners involved were described as 'not prepared to "think the unthinkable" and tried to rationalise the evidence in front of them that it did not relate to abuse' (Lock, 2013). The review stated that they lacked an 'enquiring mind' needed to perform more probing assessments, and were 'naive' about the likelihood that domestic abuse would cease, especially given that Daniel's mother had had three serial relationships with violent men and alcohol abuse was a significant problem.

Multi-agency working Following domestic violence incidents, referrals to and responses from social care were inconsistent. On some occasions assumptions were made about the actions of other agencies, and when actions were agreed at a multi-agency level, partner agencies did not ensure that these were followed up. Reassurances were made that social care was performing a core assessment, but new information was not incorporated into that assessment. Daniel's school was very concerned about his obsessive scavenging for food, and made attempts to address this with health professionals, but did not refer to social care despite identifying facial bruising. There were missed opportunities by the GP to refer to the health visitor and re-discuss concerns raised by the school. One factor which may have contributed was that the information in available hospital letters was limited (for example, no reference was made to concerns about non-accidental injury or a strategy meeting).

False reassurances Daniel's siblings appeared well cared for and Daniel was clean, not fitting the typical picture of a neglected child. There were concerns about his behaviour. He was shy, isolated, and withdrawn, and he had ritualistic behaviours and an abnormally strong bond with his older sibling. His mother was able to manipulate professionals and her portrayed image of a concerned mother was 'too readily accepted'. Daniel and his older sibling did not express any concerns about home life; however, his first language was Polish, he spoke little English, and was never spoken to directly through a formal interpreter. Also, multiple agencies inappropriately relied on his older sibling to act as an interpreter or to disclose abuse.

Inappropriate focus on the mother Despite 'Daniel being the focus of concern for all of the practitioners, in reality he was rarely the focus of their interventions'. His mother's male partners were rarely involved in enquiries or interventions, and an inappropriate level of attention was given to her ability to protect Daniel.

What can paediatricians learn from this serious case review?

At three years of age, Daniel was admitted with a spiral humeral fracture following a one-day delay in presentation. Suspicions were raised this was non-accidental injury. He was separately assessed by both paediatric and orthopaedic consultants, although the review advises that a joint assessment may have facilitated a clearer understanding of the context of injury. The elder sibling corroborated, via the police, the mechanism of accidental injury explained by the family, and at the strategy meeting the health opinion deemed the mechanism 'plausible'. This statement was deferred to as the most significant over other evidence available—for example, the delay in presentation, the other bruises, and social factors. Hence a 'rule of optimism' appeared to prevail (a tendency to positively interpret evidence, despite other available evidence to the contrary). The strategy meeting outcome was for a further social care assessment, but the collective conclusion by agencies that this was an accidental injury may have subsequently impacted on the mindset of the core assessment. The deeper analysis report (Wonnacott, 2014) recognized that the word 'plausible' could disproportionately impact on decision-making processes and it would have been more helpful to cite that both accidental and non-accidental causes were possible.

Daniel was referred by the school nurse with concerns about appetite and possible developmental delay, and was seen by a community paediatrician three weeks before he died. Previous domestic abuse history was referenced, but neither were aware of the bruises that had been seen by the school. Although his weight (0.4th percentile) and height (9–25th percentile) were measured and poor or slow weight gain was referenced, a growth chart was not completed and it was not recognized that he had lost weight. A detailed history from his mother revealed he was soiling, smearing faeces, excessively hungry, and had limited interaction at home and with peers. Together with a detailed examination, this led to concerns that this was an organic disorder and blood tests were requested (his sodium had been initially mildly raised but was in the upper range of normal on repeat). Further discussion with colleagues was planned regarding possible autistic spectrum disorder and follow-up was arranged for four months later. The review states that 'abuse was not considered as a likely differential diagnosis'. His mother's partner laughed about an incident where Daniel picked up a chip from the pavement, which should have raised further concerns about parental attitudes towards him. Daniel did not speak in the assessment. The importance of using interpreters for children whose first language is not English was highlighted as a learning point. Although previous heights and weights were recorded in the notes, the deeper analysis report (Wonnacott, 2014) subsequently found that the hospital notes were not well ordered and lacked plotted centile charts, which hampered the assessment.

What were some of the key recommendations?

Key recommendations were as follows (Lock, 2013):

- Every opportunity should be taken to protect a child and make them the focus of interventions.

- The role of the males in the family should be understood.

- Domestic violence should always be a child protection issue and the effects on the child should be examined.

- Incidents should be examined in the context of patterns of behaviour—'see the bigger picture'.

- 'Professional optimism' about a family must be supported by objective evidence.

- Height and weight should always be plotted on a growth chart.

- Abuse should be in the differential diagnosis of a child that is failing to thrive.

- Interpreters should be used where English is not the family's first language.

- Record keeping and timely reports are essential.

What other recommendations have emerged from other serious case reviews?

The most recent biennial review of serious case reviews (Brandon et al., 2012) estimated the total number of violent and maltreatment-related deaths of children (0–17 years) in England at 85 per year (1 per 100,000 children). The contribution of neglect was clearly understood for the first time, and featured in 60 per cent of serious case reviews. The national analysis highlighted the importance of strong professional supervision.

The NSPCC has summarized key recommendations from serious case reviews arranged by year or themes (NSPCC, 2014). In addition to the key recommendations from the Daniel Pelka case, you should consider the following:

- Children:
  - adopt a child-centred approach, listen to the child, and be patient and persistent in helping disengaged vulnerable children
  - recognize the warning signs of sexual exploitation and grooming.

- Family:
  - avoid reliance on mothers to protect children
  - provide opportunities for the mother to disclose in private
  - recognize disguised compliance
  - understand mental health problems in the family
  - work with adults to focus on their needs as parents, not their own individual needs.

- Substance misuse:
  - ○ analyse the misuse of alcohol or other substances and the effects on the children
  - ○ treat the self-reported quantity of consumption with caution
  - ○ regularly check that families are engaging with the support services offered.

- Professionals and agencies:
  - ○ maintain healthy scepticism and avoid 'start again syndrome'
  - ○ record domestic abuse in unambiguous language
  - ○ recognize the immediate risks to the child before implementing holistic family support packages
  - ○ prevent case 'drift' by assigning responsibility
  - ○ use the Common Assessment Framework early
  - ○ ensure adequate professional representation at meetings
  - ○ agencies must ensure adequate management and supervision, and raise awareness through training.

Conclusion

This chapter has discussed the process of serious case reviews and findings from a specific case that has some common themes with other serious case reviews nationally. Common themes that have emerged are a triad of domestic violence, alcohol and drug abuse, and mental health issues within a family. Failures of agencies to share information and not trusting parents' word without speaking to the child are amongst the most valuable lessons to be learned.

References

Brandon, M., Sidebotham, P., Bailey, S. and Belderson, P. (2011). *A Study of Recommendations Arising from Serious Case Reviews 2009 to 2010*, Research Report DFE-RR157, Department for Education. Available at: http://www.gov.uk/government/uploads/system/uploads/attachment_data/file/182521/DFE-RR157.pdf (accessed 15 July 2010).

Brandon, M., Sidebotham, P., Bailey, S. et al. (2012). *New learning from serious case reviews: a two year report for 2009–2011*. Research Report DFE-RR226. Available at: http://www.uea.ac.uk/centre-research-child-family/child-protection-and-family-support/new-learning-from-scrs (accessed 15 July 2015).

HM Government (2006). *The Local Safeguarding Children Boards Regulations*. Available at: http://www.legislation.gov.uk/uksi/2006/90/pdfs/uksi_20060090_en.pdf (accessed 15 July 2015).

HM Government (2010). *Working Together to Safeguard Children: A Guide to Inter-agency Working to Safeguard and Promote the Welfare of Children*. Available at: http://webarchive. nationalarchives.gov.uk/20130401151715/https://www.education.gov.uk/publications/ eorderingdownload/00305-2010dom-en-v3.pdf (accessed 15 July 2015).

HM Government (2015). *Working Together to Safeguard Children: A Guide to Inter-agency Working to Safeguard and Promote the Welfare of Children*. Available at: https://www.gov.uk/ government/uploads/system/uploads/attachment_data/file/419595/Working_Together_to_ Safeguard_Children.pdf (accessed 15 July 2015).

Lock, R. (2013). *Coventry LSCB—Final Overview Report of Serious Case Review re Daniel Pelka*. Available at: http://www.coventrylscb.org.uk/dpelka.html (accessed 19 January 2014).

Munro E. (2011). *The Munro Review of Child Protection: Final Report—A Child-Centred System*. London: TSO.

NSPCC (National Society for the Prevention of Cruelty to Children) (2014). *At-a-Glance Thematic Briefings—Learning from Case Reviews*. Available at: http://www.nspcc.org.uk/ Inform/resourcesforprofessionals/scrs/at-a-glance-briefings_wda99475.html (accessed 19 January 2014).

R v Mariusz Krezolek and Magdelena Luczak [2013]. T20127199, Birmingham Crown Court. Sentencing remarks of Mrs Justice Cox.

Wonnacott, J. (2014). *Daniel Pelka Review: Deeper Analysis and Progress Report on Implementation of Recommendations*. Available at: http://www.coventrylscb.org.uk/dpelka.html (accessed 12 June 2014).

22

Child protection in low-resource settings

Christopher Hands

Chapter summary

Child maltreatment is a global public health problem. A recent meta-analysis of studies on childhood physical abuse (Stoltenborgh et al., 2013) showed a combined prevalence from self-report studies of 22.6 per cent, and the prevalence figures did not differ significantly by region or by ethnicity of the group studied. A large proportion of children are maltreated in all regions and cultures across the world. In many countries fewer resources are available for the detection and management of child maltreatment, and doctors working in these settings may face different challenges to those working in the UK. This chapter describes some of these challenges, outlines resources that may be available, and suggests strategies for keeping children safe in low-resource settings. The cases are based on personal experience in the regions described, and therefore are limited to Africa, but could be applied to other low-resource settings in general terms.

Case 22.1 Working in emergency protection environments

You are the paediatrician in a hospital in the Dadaab refugee camps in Northeast Kenya. Eight-year-old Faiza is carried in by her aunt. Faiza's lower face and chest are covered with partial-thickness burns which look like splash marks. Whilst you administer pain relief and dress the burns, her aunt tells you that Faiza's mother became cross when she discovered that Faiza had been playing with her friends and had not fetched water as she had been asked. Once Faiza has been admitted to the ward, you ask her aunt to tell you more about the situation at home. There are seven other children in their dwelling, and Faiza's mother has been extremely stressed since her husband left. The aunt is finding it difficult to know how to talk to her about the situation.

Case 22.1 Exercise

◆ What are Faiza's rights and what is their legal basis?

◆ What local frameworks and systems for protecting children may exist in settings where there are few resources?

◆ What can you do to ensure that Faiza's brothers and sisters are safe?

Case 22.1 Discussion

What are Faiza's rights and what is their legal basis?

The UN Convention on the Rights of the Child (UNICEF, 1989) defines the rights of children everywhere, and has been ratified by every country in the world apart from the USA, Somalia, and the Republic of South Sudan. It was ratified by the UK in 1991. All States Parties to the convention are required to make regular submissions to the UN Committee on the Rights of the Child (CRC) to describe the systems that are in place within the country to uphold children's rights, and what work is being undertaken to improve them. Article 19.1 of the Convention states that:

> Parties shall take all appropriate legislative, administrative, social and educational measures to protect the child from all forms of physical or mental violence, injury or abuse, neglect or negligent treatment, maltreatment or exploitation, including sexual abuse, while in the care of parent(s), legal guardian(s) or any other person who has the care of the child.

What local frameworks and systems for protecting children may exist in settings where there are few resources?

The shelter, food, healthcare, and sanitation services at the Dadaab refugee camps are provided by the UN High Commission for Refugees (UNHCR) and its partners. UNHCR has a child protection framework which is publicly available (UNHCR, 2012), and various agencies deliver child protection services within the camps. The largest such agency is Save the Children, whose services are organized around child welfare committees whose members are community and religious leaders. In many emergency protection situations such as refugee camps, safeguarding structures are increasingly put in place early on, and it is always important to investigate what services are available.

What can you do to ensure that Faiza's brothers and sisters are safe?

There are other children in the house who may be at risk of harm. In such situations it is common for other members of the extended family to take care of the children for a period. Faiza's aunt has brought her to the hospital, and it would be appropriate to enquire as to whether she or other members of the family may be able to look after the children. If that is not possible, a representative of the local child welfare committee would be able to investigate what temporary care might be possible.

Case 22.2 Children outside normal protection structures

You are working in a paediatric clinic on the outskirts of Khartoum, run by a medical relief agency. Twelve-year-old Noor walks in the door of the clinic, bleeding from a ragged 10 cm laceration to his left cheek. You stitch and dress the wound; Noor stares straight ahead during the procedure and does not look at you. When you have finished you ask one of your Sudanese colleagues to help you to take a history. Your colleague is reluctant to help you, but eventually attends and interprets as you ask questions of Noor. He is brusque in his interactions with the child. Noor has been living on the street for more than a year; he begs and occasionally steals. Tonight he got into an argument with one of the older boys who 'wanted to hurt him'. The older boy cut his face with a broken bottle. Noor then asks you for money to buy food. Your colleague tells you to 'Send him out—he shouldn't be here anymore'.

Case 22.2 Exercise

- What other risks does Noor face?

- What support might you be able to offer Noor?

- How might you address your colleague's attitude towards Noor's situation?

Case 22.2 Discussion

What other risks does Noor face?

Children who have the street as a central reference point in their lives are exposed to multiple risks. In addition to the risk of physical violence from other children, street children are at risk of violence from many adults, including some in responsible positions, such as police officers (Thomas de Benitez, 2007). They are also exposed to a high risk of sexual violence on the part of adults or other children. They risk exposure and addiction to intoxicant drugs, commonly solvents. Many children connected to the street are involved in some of the worst forms of child labour, including commercial sex work, as described in the UNHCR Worst Forms of Child Labour Convention (1999).

What support might you be able to offer to Noor?

Across the world there are many organizations working with street-connected children. These organizations commonly provide night shelters, counselling, and informal education provision. Many employ street educators who provide support and advice to children in the street at night. There is often not a list of these and similar organizations in hospital emergency departments, and it is worthwhile putting together a list of such agencies. In many settings, a network of non-governmental organizations delivers the child protection system on the ground, without significant involvement from the national government. In low-resource settings, it is often important to develop your own network of contacts which can be used in urgent situations.

How might you address your colleague's attitude towards Noor's situation?

Children living on the street are the victims of discrimination in many countries. A UN High Commissioner for Human Rights report identifies the most complex challenge faced by street children as 'dealing with the perceptions of those around them and the treatment they are consequently afforded' (UNHCHR, 2012). Other groups of children face similar perceptions and prejudices, such as disabled children or those with particular health problems such as epilepsy or albinism. Confronting the prejudices of those with whom you work is difficult, and must be undertaken slowly and with great sensitivity. Nevertheless, one of the most useful and achievable goals in international child protection is to build a non-judgemental, robust, and unified approach to child protection in one institution. There are many ways to approach this, and some widely used tools are published by Keeping Children Safe (http://www.keepingchildrensafe.org.uk/resources).

Case 22.3 Children at risk of harm from traditional practices

You are working in a small clinic in a rural area of Uganda. You go into the nurse's room to get some supplies; when you enter a child who looks about three years old is about to be given an immunization. You notice that there are several distinct circular burns of varying ages across her buttocks. The child's mother does not look at or speak to you. After the child and mother have left the room, you go back in to speak to the nurse. She explains that the burns are part of a traditional treatment, and that the child's mother was reluctant to engage with you because a previous European doctor at the clinic had 'tried to make trouble for her'.

Case 22.3 Exercise

♦ What strategies are available to you to combat the harm being done to this child?

♦ What lessons can be drawn from the actions of your predecessor?

Case 22.3 Discussion

What strategies are available to you to combat the harm being done to the child?

Traditional remedies are often used instead of biomedical treatments because traditional healers draw on shared cultural knowledge and experience to explain their treatments, can be found closer to home, and may offer their treatments at cheaper prices than medicines (Rutebemberwa et al., 2013). They may also often fill a gap, as supplies of medicines may frequently run out in rural clinics. It is not possible to change all of these factors, but it may be possible to persuade patients to choose biomedical treatments alongside traditional treatments and to reduce any harm from those traditional remedies. In this case, it is clear that the child's mother is still willing to engage with biomedical treatments, as she has brought her child to be immunized. If possible, it would be helpful to ask the clinic nurse if she could discuss the reason why the burning has been performed with the child's mother, and to explore whether the child has another health problem which needs investigation. At a further appointment it might be possible to address the health risks posed by the burns.

What lessons can be drawn from the actions of your predecessor?

In many low-resource settings, child protection systems have been imposed by outside agencies with little regard for local traditions, which has left those communities feeling that their practices and resources have been disrespected and marginalized (Save the Children, 2009). Changes in child protection practices have been most successfully implemented where they have been built on, and in partnership with, existing community structures. In seeking to protect a child, it is possible to do more harm than good by trying to impose new expectations and structures without a period of consultation and discussion.

Conclusion

Child maltreatment is just as common in poor countries as in rich ones. In many of those countries there are few resources at hand, and sometimes those working with children need to find pragmatic solutions to ensure the safety of the children they meet. However, there are often many resources available and structures in place to help keep children safe in difficult circumstances. UK doctors working overseas should apprise themselves early of relevant local organizations and guidelines, preferably before departure. You will encounter child protection cases; it is clearly better to know what approach you would take before the child is in front of you.

References

Rutebemberwa, E., Lubega, M., Katureeba, K.S., Oundo, A., Kiweewa, F., Mukanga, D.(2013). Use of traditional medicine for the treatment of diabetes in Eastern Uganda: a qualitative exploration of reasons for choice. *BMC International Health and Human Rights*, **13**(1).

Save the Children. (2009). *What Are We Learning About Protecting Children in the Community?* Available at: http://www.savethechildren.org.uk/resources/online-library/what-are-we-learning-about-protecting-children-in-the-community (accessed 15 July 2015).

Stoltenburgh, M., Bakermans-Kranenburg, M.J., Van Ijzendoorn, M.H., Alink, L.R.A. (2013). Cultural–geographical differences in the occurrence of child physical abuse? A meta-analysis of global prevalence. *International Journal of Psychology*, **48**(2), 81–94.

Thomas de Benitez, S. (2007). *State of the World's Street Children: Violence*. Available at: http://www.streetchildrenresources.org/resources/state-of-the-worlds-street-children-violence/ (accessed 15 July 2015).

UNHCHR (UN High Commissioner for Human Rights). (2012). *Report of the United Nations High Commissioner for Human Rights on the Protection and Promotion of the Rights of Children Working and/or Living on the Street*. Geneva: United Nations.

UNHCR (UN High Commissioner for Refugees). (2012). *A Framework for the Protection of Children*. Geneva: United Nations.

UNICEF (UN International Children's Emergency Fund). (1989). *Convention on the Rights of the Child*. Geneva: United Nations.

Appendix 1

Social care referral guidance and example

Gayle Hann

Guidance when making social care referrals

♦ Fill out the referral form as fully as possible ensuring that you have the correct name, date of birth, and address of the child. Explore information that is not readily available with the family, such as name and dates of birth for both parents and anyone else who may be significant or live in the household, including siblings and any school or nursery that they may attend.

♦ State clearly why you are making the referral; for example 'I am making this referral as I am concerned that the child has been physically abused'.

♦ Describe as clearly and thoroughly as possible what happened that has led to safeguarding concerns and list your evidence for coming to this conclusion/ assessment.

♦ Do not use medical terminology or jargon.

♦ Ensure that you have referred the child to the correct social care department; this is particularly important in hospitals that border with many boroughs/counties.

♦ Where a child or family indicates that they have a current social worker, elicit the details of the worker and the local authority that they work for and send your referral to that authority.

♦ If the family have recently moved house, it is useful to ask for their previous address as the family may not be known to the local social care department but may be known elsewhere.

♦ All referrals must include the NHS number for the child to comply with new National Health Service Child Protection Information Service (NHS CP-IS) requirements—this is a new computer system which was introduced in a few leading boroughs in November 2014.

◆ **CONSENT**: Parents/child should be informed of a social care referral unless doing so puts the child at further risk. If this is a child in need, you must gain consent. This means that if you believe that the child is NOT at immediate risk of harm, but would benefit from some support services as a child in need, you must gain consent for information sharing and services from the child/parent/carer BEFORE making the referral.

◆ Always follow up verbal referrals with a written referral (email/fax is usually satisfactory if acknowledged) as soon as possible.

◆ It is essential that any personal information about families should be treated with the utmost confidentiality and security. For this reason, information about families, including your referral, should not be sent through unsecured email, but should be sent to a secure email account (for social care this will have a GSI/GCSX suffix) from your nhs.net account.

Please note that the referral that follows is an example and different social care departments use different forms, such as the Common Assessment Framework (CAF), and may ask for different information. The example given is that of the child in Case 2.1 from Chapter 2. You may want to read this case before reading the referral form that follows.

Example of a social care referral form

Remember—if your request is urgent, you should contact the relevant team by phone immediately, and then complete and send this form by secure e-mail within 24 hours.

If this form is sent confirming an earlier phone referral, please state the date of your call, and the name of the person you spoke to:
Name of person spoken to: Nigel Bowers
Date of phone call: 25/02/14

1. Details of child/ren/young person referred

Child/ren/young person's name/s:

Family Name:	Forename:
Davies	Jasmine

Also known as:
Ask whether the child is known by any other name.

Date of birth/expected date of delivery: 11/08/2008   Gender: Female

Home address:	Phone number:
12 Cherry Tree Avenue, Walthamstow, London	02083456789
Postcode: E17 9BU	07791234567

Previous address:
14 Maybush Avenue, Barnet, Hertfordshire
Postcode: EN4 3NW

On Child Protection Register? No

Child/ren's/young person's first language: English

Child/ren's/young person's preferred means of communication: English

Interpreter/signer required: No

Child/young person's religion: Christian	Child/young person's nationality: British

Disability/special educational needs:
None

2. Details of parents/main carers

Mother's name: Rosemary Davies	
Date of birth/Age: 01/01/1984	
Ethnicity: White British	
Language: English	Interpreter/signer required: No
Father's name: Matthew Davies	
Date of birth: 01/01/1982	
Ethnicity: White British	
Language: English	Interpreter/signer required: No

3. Other children in the family/household

Name	Address	Age	Gender	School
Thomas Davies (brother)	As above	18 mths	M	
Isabel Davies (sister)	As above	9 yrs	F	St Botolph's C of E Primary

4. Key Professionals/Agencies

	Name	Phone no.		Name	Phone no.
Health visitor/ school nurse			Asylum team		
GP/ community paediatrician	Dr Ansari Park Medical Centre, Walthamstow, London E17 9BU	0208345678	Substance misuse services		
School/ nursery	Cherry Tree Primary School, Walthamstow, London E17 9BU	0208123455	Hospital/ Consultant/ ward	Dr Jane Evans Paediatric Consultant, Walthamstow Hospital, London E17 9BU	0208871234

Education welfare		Social Services Team		
Police		Youth Offending Team		
Community mental health/ CAMHS		Other		

5. Referrer details

Name: Rina Choudhary

Position: ST4 paeds doctor

Address: Walthamstow Hospital	Phone number: 0208812345
Postcode: E17 9BU	

Date of referral: 25/02/2014

NHS net email account: rchoudhary235@nhs.net	Date: 25/02/2014

6. Reason for referral

What are your concerns about this child/children/young person? *If making an allegation of abuse, please give specific details, with dates, times, details of any witnesses, and explanations given.*

Reason for referral:

Possible physical and emotional abuse

Jasmine presented to the Emergency Department on 25/02/2014 with a four-month history of intermittent abdominal pain. During her examination, it was noted that she had a small circular bruise to her left ear which is suspected to be a result of non-accidental injury as this is an unusual injury. Her nine-year-old sister, Isabel, was also noted to have a black eye which was reported to have been caused when her 18-month-old brother, Thomas, threw a beaker at her. I am not satisfied with this explanation and suspect that this may also be an abusive injury. Jasmine has not spoken at all during her assessment at the hospital, but her mother reports that she can talk. Neither Jasmine nor Isabel have made any statements about how these injuries have been caused but both looked to their mother when asked.

Jasmine is having investigations for her abdominal pain, but all investigations so far have been normal and a psychological cause for her pain is being considered.

7. Supporting information

7.1 Child's developmental needs and identified risk factors

(Please comment on the information you have about health, emotional and behavioural development, education, identity, family and social relationships, social presentation, and self care.)

Family previously known to social services for domestic violence (father to mother). Parents still live in same household—possible ongoing domestic violence. The family moved to this area six months ago.

At the time of attendance at hospital the children were clean and dressed appropriately for the weather, but presented as shy or withdrawn. Neither Jasmine nor Isabel responded to my efforts to engage them in conversation and both appeared reluctant to maintain eye contact with me.

7.2 Specific issues affecting parenting

(Please comment on the information you have about basic care, emotional warmth/ stimulation, ensuring safety, guidance and boundaries, substance misuse, domestic violence, housing.)

Jasmine did not seem worried about being left on her own on the ward when her mother took her other two children home. Although her mother has appropriately brought her to the Emergency Department for recurrent abdominal pain, Jasmine does not seem to have a particularly close relationship with her mother, as evidenced by her mother stating that Jasmine is 'a difficult child who does not do as she is told'.

7.3 Other factors that affect the child

(Please comment on information you have about family history, wider family/community support, cultural considerations relevant to an assessment of the child's needs, income, other issues affecting the child/ren.)

8. Consent for information storage and information sharing

Parents/carers, children, and young people must give their explicit consent for information to be shared with other agencies in order to support need and offer additional services.

The only exception to this is where you have child protection concerns that reach the threshold for compulsory intervention and consent has been denied or seeking consent may jeopardize the welfare of the child or young person.

Parent and/or **Child/Young Person** (delete where appropriate) understands that the information recorded on this form will be stored and used for the purpose of providing services to the family.

Explicit consent has been obtained for information being shared with and/or a referral being made to agency/agencies as necessary. ☒ Yes

There are statutory grounds for sharing this information without consent? **N/A**

Appendix 2

Child protection medical assessment

Gayle Hann

Child's name	
Date of birth	
Sex	
Ethnicity	
Address	
Primary carers	
Person with parental responsibility	
GP	
Health visitor/school nurse	
School/nursery	
Long-term social worker	
Child protection plan/court order	
Date of assessment	
Time of assessment	
Assessment requested by:	
Interpreter used	
Persons present (name and telephone number): 1. 2. 3.	
Social worker and contact details	
Police name and contact number	
Examining doctor and GMC number	

Consent for child protection medical assessment

I give my consent for:

1.	medical examination	Y/N
2.	relevant investigations (e.g. blood tests, X-rays)	Y/N
3.	photography of clinical findings for patient records	Y/N
4.	medical report to be shared with GP, health visitor/ school nurse, social care, and police.	Y/N

I give permission for photographs to be used:

1.	for teaching/training purposes	Y/N
2.	for peer review	Y/N
3.	to support clinical evidence in court proceedings.	Y/N

Parent/carer

Name: Relationship to child:

Signed: Date:

Child (where applicable)

Name:

Signed: Date:

Doctor

Name:

Signed: Date:

Information from referrer

History of the incident from parent/carer

History from the child and child's views

Use his or her own words.

Alone or in the presence of:

Current health status

Systemic enquiry including diet and sleep.

Behaviour

Conduct (withdrawn, disruptive, aggressive, sexualized, etc.), wetting, soiling, self-harm, bullying, substance abuse, alcohol, tobacco use.

Past medical history

Birth history:

Medical history:

Previous A&E attendances and hospital admissions:

Date	Hospital	Presenting problem	Notes available

Medications and allergies:

Immunizations:

Development

Provide details of milestones. Provide adequate details regarding mobility of the child if unexplained injuries. Consideration should be given to a detailed developmental review.

Nursery/school

Attendance, progress, extra help, special needs, statement of educational needs.

Menstrual and sexual health

Where applicable.

Specific questions for a child presenting with bruising

	Yes	No	Details
Birth history of bleeding (e.g. umbilical cord bleeding or cephalohaematoma)			
History of bleeding: ◆ spontaneous prolonged epistaxis ◆ after surgery or dental extraction ◆ with IM injections ◆ menorrhagia			
Drug history: ◆ NSAIDs ◆ anticoagulation ◆ steroids			
Family history: ◆ bleeding disorder ◆ Excessive bleeding surgery/dental extractions			

Specific questions for a child presenting with a fracture

	Yes	No	Details
Family history of fractures			
Family history of deafness			
Family history of dental problems			
Maternal vitamins in pregnancy			
Infant feeding			
Infant supplements			

Family and social history

Family composition (genogram)

Primary carer: Name: Date of Birth:

Marital status	
Relationship to child	
Ethnic group	
Country of birth	
Language spoken	
Occupation	
Health	
Mental health	
Alcohol, drugs, smoking	
Domestic violence	

Second carer: Name: Date of birth:

Marital status	
Relationship to child	
Ethnic group	
Country of birth	
Language spoken	
Occupation	
Health	
Mental health	
Alcohol, drugs, smoking	
Domestic violence	

Other significant adults

Financial/housing and any other relevant family/social information

Examination

Persons present during the examination:

Weight:	(centile)	Head circumference:	(centile)
Height/length:	(centile)	BMI:	(centile)

General observation

Emotional state, demeanour and interactions, parent–child interactions.

General condition

Clothes

Cleanliness

Hair and nails

Nappies/rash

Infestation

Pallor

Mouth: upper and lower frenula, teeth

Ears

CVS, RS, GI, CNS

Anus/genitalia

Tanner staging

Abnormalities noted on the skin

List injuries noting size, shape, colour, site of injury, any explanations offered for each:

Number of body maps used:

Photography: Y/N

Investigations

Investigation	Yes	Where done	Date	Result	Action
X-ray					
Skeletal survey					
CT head					
MRI head					
Hb, WCC, platelets, film					
Clotting studies					
Bone profile					
LFTs and amylase					
Vitamin D and PTH					
Other					

Summary

Risk factors

Medical opinion

Discussed with paediatric consultant Dr:

Consider accidental explanations, medical explanations for findings, whether injury may be non-accidental, other forms of abuse (emotional, sexual, neglect).

Unmet medical needs

For example, dentist, developmental assessment, CAMHS referral, sexual health.

Need	Action required	Done by

Recommendations and follow-up

Signed:

Date:

Appendix 3

Format for a statement to court

Karen Aucott

Often, your court report will be similar/identical to your medical report (civil) (See Chapter 15, Case 15.3, for how to write a medical report) or police statement (criminal) (see Appendix 4). In criminal cases, you will often be asked to clarify or consider further or certain elements of your evidence. The Child Abuse Investigation Unit may ask you to respond to questions frequently asked by the Crown Prosecution Service in similar cases; it is best to respond to each question in turn and to explain more complex medical terms in lay language.

Strictly confidential

I, Dr Lucy Smith, am a paediatric registrar working at the Moonstrike Hospital in Northumbria. My qualifications are MBChB and MRCPCH. I have been working within paediatrics for ten years and have been carrying out child protection medicals for the past four years.

On 29 January 2014, I was the paediatric registrar on call when Joseph Lloyd, a four-month-old boy, presented to the children's emergency department having had an acute episode of high-pitched crying with subsequent floppiness and laboured breathing. He had been unwell for the previous 24 hours with cold-like symptoms and had not been feeding as well as usual. Otherwise his parents had not noticed anything unusual. Investigations revealed multiple subdural haemorrhages (bleeds around the brain) and extensive bilateral retinal haemorrhages (bleeds to the back of the eye). My medical report, which you have previously received, concluded that these injuries were highly suggestive of non-accidental head injury (previously known as shaken baby syndrome).

Many thanks for your request for further information which I am happy to assist with.

How did your clinical reasoning lead you to conclude that non-accidental head injury was the most likely cause of Joseph's injuries?

The combination of subdural haemorrhages, retinal haemorrhages, and an associated change in neurological status (such as an altered level of consciousness, floppiness, breathing difficulty, or seizures) are commonly seen in non-accidental head injury (see Box A3.1). All of these features were present in Joseph's case and no alternative explanations have been given to account for the injuries.

Box A3.1 Evidence base

In children under the age of three, when intracranial haemorrhages and retinal haemorrhages are present together, the probability that the child has sustained a non-accidental head injury is 71 per cent (OR 3.5).

More information can be found at: Cardiff Child Protection Systematic reviews 2013. *Core Info.* http://core-info.cardiff.ac.uk.

Reproduced from *Archives of Disease in Childhood*, 94 (11), S. Maguire, N. Pickerd, D. Farewell, M. Mann, V. Tempest, and A. M. Kemp, Which clinical features distinguish inflicted from non-inflicted brain injury? A systematic review, pp. 860–867, doi:10.1136/adc.2008.150110, (c) 2009, BMJ Publishing Group Ltd. With permission from BMJ Publishing Group Ltd.

Alternative medical causes of subdural haemorrhages/retinal haemorrhages were considered.

The child did not have a temperature and there were no laboratory markers of infection. Whilst intracranial infections can cause subdural haemorrhages, associated retinal haemorrhages are not commonly seen. Joseph's clotting studies were within the normal range. Examination did not reveal any associated bruises and there was no previous personal or family history of easy bruising or bleeding.

At times, changes to the sodium salt levels in the body can cause subdural haemorrhages. Joseph's sodium level was within the normal range.

There were no clinical features to suggest a metabolic problem.

Is it possible to identify the date that the injury was caused?

Joseph presented after an acute episode of high-pitched crying and it is possible that a shaking injury occurred shortly before this; the sudden silence, subsequent floppiness, and laboured breathing are likely to be a consequence of the bleed into the head. The radiological report does not suggest a time frame for the bleed.

For further information/comment on radiological studies, you will need to contact the reporting neuroradiologist.

Can a mechanism for causing the injuries be identified?

It is commonly accepted that non-accidental head injury results from severe repetitive shaking, but I would refer you to an expert witness for more detail on the mechanisms.

Assuming that the injury was caused by shaking, can you articulate the severity of the shaking or the length of time that the shaking lasted?

Considerable force would be needed whilst shaking a baby to cause subdural haemorrhages and retinal haemorrhages—these are not findings which are associated with routine care or playful bouncing or jumping around with a baby.

I am not able to comment on the length of time that the child would have been shaken for to account for these injuries.

Could the injuries have occurred without any physical signs being apparent to the caregiver?

A child who has been shaken with sufficient force to cause subdural haemorrhages and retinal haemorrhages is likely to have shown some physical signs (as well as being distressed at the time of the incident) but, depending on the size of the bleed, these signs may have been subtle, such as lethargy and poor feeding.

Could earlier medical treatment have resulted in less permanent damage to the child?

At the current time, I am not able to predict the child's long-term prognosis or whether earlier intervention would have resulted in a different prognosis.

Please do not hesitate to contact me if you require any further assistance.

Yours sincerely,

Dr Lucy Smith

Paediatric Registrar, ST6

Appendix 4

Guidance on completing a police statement and example of a police statement

Gayle Hann

When making a police statement, ensure accuracy by reviewing your notes to make certain that there are no discrepancies between the medical notes and your statement. When making your statement, consider the following guidance.

- To avoid inappropriate disclosure of addresses to the defence, do not write your own or the patient's address on the front of the statement.

- Start the statement with your employment and qualifications; for example, 'I am employed as a doctor at (name and address of hospital/surgery). My qualifications are . . . '.

- State when and where you performed the examination; for example, 'On day, date, time, and place, and with consent, I examined (patient's name and date of birth)'.

- State the reason for examination; for example, 'Section 47 medical examination for alleged assault by . . . '.

- Say what your examination findings are; for example, 'On examination I found . . . ' (give full details of examination findings in both medical and layman's terms).

- State whether you think that the history is consistent with the examination findings.

- State any treatment required or given.

♦ In serious assault cases, your opinion as to any probable long-term prognosis may be appropriate; for example, in head injuries state whether you think that it may impact on the child's development.

♦ If you refer to any diagrams or body maps, they should be attached with consecutive numbering and should be originals and not photocopies (as in Chapter 17, Figures 17.5 and 17.6).

♦ Your full details should be included at the back of the statement with any dates to avoid for court.

This guidance is adapted from guidance by the Metropolitan Police on how to fill out a witness statement.

WITNESS STATEMENT

CJ Act 1967, s.9; MC Act 1980, ss.5A(3)(a) and 5B; Criminal Procedure Rules 2005, Rule 27.1

Statement of	Dr Gayle Hann	URN:
Age if under 18 (if over 18 insert 'over 18')	Occupation:	Medical doctor

This statement (consisting of: **2** pages each signed by me) is true to the best of my knowledge and belief and I make it knowing that, if it is tendered in evidence, I shall be liable to prosecution if I have wilfully stated anything in it which I know to be false, or do not believe to be true.

Signature:		Date:	04/09/2014
Tick if witness evidence is visually recorded	☐	(supply witness details on rear)	

My name is Dr Gayle Hann. I am employed as a paediatric doctor and have been working for the community paediatric team as a specialist registrar at the North London Hospital NHS Trust, Goldthorn Way, N16 1QX, since September 2013. I qualified in medicine from Sheffield University in August 2002. My qualifications are MBChB and I am a member of the Royal College of Paediatrics and Child Health.

I was the community doctor on duty on Friday, 4 September 2014 at 10.00 hours when Isabel Clark was brought to St Mark's Community Hospital for a Section 47 child protection medical by social worker Anwa Appadoo and DC Jude Hends (see Chapter 17).

I was given the history that on 2 September 2014, Isabel Clark, aged nine years old (date of birth: 14 May 2005), had accompanied her six-year-old sister,

Jasmine, to the hospital. Jasmine had been suffering from abdominal pain and had been found to have a bruise to her left ear. During the course of the examination, child protection concerns were raised. Isabel had been noted to have a bruise to her right eye. Isabel's mother did not accompany her today to explain what had happened to her right eye, but on 2 September 2014 had informed the A&E doctor on duty that Isabel had sustained a black eye when her two-year-old brother had thrown a beaker in her face. I was able to contact Isabel's mother over the phone and she repeated this history. Isabel is an otherwise fit and well girl who has no other medical problems and takes no medications.

I examined Isabel today (4 September 2014 at 10.00 hours) and recorded any injuries on a body map.

Examination

Isabel was dressed in clean but well-worn clothes. She was on the 25th centile for growth. She had a shy demeanour and avoided direct eye contact. Her hair was clean, but the nails on her hands and feet were dirty. She had a normal examination apart from the marks documented on body maps 1 and 2 (see Chapter 17).

Mark 1

Isabel's right eye was bruised and swollen shut. The swelling and bruising of her right eye was 4 × 4.5 cm in size with a 0.8 × 0.1 cm laceration through the right eyebrow.

I asked the following question and have documented Isabel's response verbatim:

Dr Hann: 'Isabel, what happened to your eye?'

Isabel: 'Daddy punched me.'

Mark 2

Isabel had a 2 × 3 cm graze to her left knee which had scabbed over.

I asked the following question and have documented Isabel's response verbatim:

Dr Hann: 'Isabel, what happened to your knee?'

Isabel: 'I fell over in the playground at school.'

Marks 3 and 4

Isabel had a 1 × 1 cm bruise and a 1 × 2 cm bruise beneath mark 3 to her left shin.

I asked the following question and have documented Isabel's response verbatim:

Dr Hann: 'Isabel, what happened to your leg?'

Isabel: 'I can't remember. . . . I think I caught it on my bike pedal last week.'

Mark 5

Isabel had a 4 × 6 cm bluish mark to her lower back.

I asked the following question and have documented Isabel's response verbatim:

Dr Hann: 'Isabel, do you know what this bluish mark is on your back?'

Isabel: 'I have always had it. . . . Mummy told me it is a birthmark.'

None of Isabel's injuries required any treatment, but I have referred her to Moorfield's Eye Hospital to rule out a significant eye injury as she was unable to open her eye.

Medical opinion

Mark 1, the bruise and laceration to her right eye, was most likely caused by non-accidental injury. The explanation given by Isabel's mother, that it was caused by Isabel's two-year-old brother throwing a cup, is not consistent with the injury. Isabel's right eye injury is unlikely to be caused by her brother, as a toddler is unlikely to be able to generate enough force to cause such an injury. Marks 2–4 on the legs are common in active children and are consistent with the explanation given; therefore they are likely to be accidental in nature. Mark 5 is probably a birthmark.

Case summary

In my medical opinion, Isabel has suffered significant harm and it is highly likely that she has been the victim of physical abuse by her father, based on my examination and Isabel's own disclosure that her father punched her.

Appendix 5

Brief guidelines on chain of evidence

Gayle Hann

The chain of evidence is a legal concept which requires that the origin and history of any specimen that may later be produced as evidence in court must be clearly demonstrated to have had an unbroken chain from its source to the court (Thomas et al., 2002).

- A chain of evidence form should be used to clearly document who has taken the sample.

- The person taking the sample should keep the sample in their possession, and all persons who handle the sample should be clearly documented with time, place, date, and signatures as appropriate.

- Problems typically arise when the need to start a chain of evidence is not appreciated.

- One form must be used for each specimen.

- Full guidance on the taking and handling of forensic samples can be found in the document *National Guidelines on a Standardised Proforma for 'Chain of Evidence' Specimen Collection and on the Retention and Storage of Specimens Relating to the Management of Suspected Sexually Transmitted Infections in Children and Young People* (RCP, 2005).

Chain of evidence form

A copy of this form must accompany specimens associated with medico-legal investigations or where documentation is required for audit purposes.
All specimens and related documentation MUST remain within the custody of the appropriate signatory at all times.

Specimen Collection and Transportation

PATIENT DETAILS	
Hospital number:	Date of examination:
Surname:	Examining doctor:
First name:	Designation:
Date of birth:	Signature:
Relevant patient information:	

SPECIMEN DETAILS	
Taken by:	Date taken:
Designation:	Time taken:
Signature:	Type of specimen:

Individuals entrusted with the custody of the specimen and form during transportation to the laboratory must complete the section below. If transfer of custody is necessary the next available section must be completed by the new custodian in the presence of the previous bearer. The same procedure must be followed when the specimen is handed over to laboratory personnel.

TRANSPORTATION DETAILS (specimen custodians)			
1.	Name:	Date:	Time:
	Designation:		
	Signature:		
2.	Name:	Date:	Time:
	Designation:		
	Signature:		
3.	Name:	Date:	Time:
	Designation:		
	Signature:		

4.	Name:	Date:	Time:
	Designation:		
	Signature:		

Sample Laboratory Chain of Evidence Form

Lab no:	Date received:	Time received:
Patient's details: Surname: Forename: Date of birth:	Specimen type:	
Doctor's name: Signature:	Specimen taken by: Signature:	
Specimen taken to the laboratory by: Signature:		

Work on this specimen should be performed or directly supervised, by one BMS 2/3. If this responsibility is passed on to another BMS 3/4, they should satisfy themselves that the tests performed relate to the correct specimen, and then sign and put the date and time on the form below.

	Print name	Signature	Date	Time
Received by BMS: Y/N				
Handed over to BMS: 2/3 Y/N				
Consultant check of interim report: Y/N Organisms to save: Y/N				
Consultant check of interim report: Y/N Organisms to save: Y/N				
Date of interim report:		Date of final report:		

Staple this form to the request card. After work on the specimen has been completed, file both in the designated file in the laboratory manager's office.
NB: All names must be accompanied by a signature.

References

Royal College of Pathologists. (2005). *National Guidelines on a Standardised Proforma for 'Chain of Evidence' Specimen Collection and on the Retention and Storage of Specimens Relating to the Management of Suspected Sexually Transmitted Infections in Children and Young People*. Available at: http://www.rcpath.org/Resources/RCPath/Migrated%20Resources/ Documents/C/ChainOfEvidence-June06.pdf (accessed 1 November 2014.

Thomas, A., Forster, G., Robinson, A., Rogstad, K. (2002) National guideline on the management of suspected sexually transmitted infections in children and young people. *Sexually Transmitted Infections* 78, 324–31.

Appendix 6

Body maps

Conrad von Stempel

1. Baby AP (anteroposterior)

2. Baby PA (posteroanterior)

3. Baby left lateral

4. Baby right lateral

5. Toddler AP (anteroposterior)

6. Toddler PA (posteroanterior)

7. Toddler left lateral

8. Toddler right lateral

9. Young male child AP (anteroposterior)

10. Young male child PA (posteroanterior)

11. Young male child left lateral

12. Young male child right lateral

13. Young female child AP (anteroposterior)

14. Young female child PA (posteroanterior)

15. Young female child left lateral

16. Young female child right lateral

17. Male teenager AP (anteroposterior)

18. Male teenager PA (posteroanterior)

19. Male teenager left lateral

20. Male teenager right lateral

21. Female teenager AP (anteroposterior)

22. Female teenager PA (posteroanterior)

23. Female teenager left lateral

24. Female teenager right lateral

25. Scalp (skyline view)

26. Eyes

27. Frenuli

28. Left ear

29. Right ear

30. Left hand and axilla

31. Right hand and axilla

32. Male and female genitalia

33. Feet dorsal surface

34. Feet plantar surface

Patient Name:
Hospital Number:
NHS Number:
Date of Birth:
Date of Examination:
Examiner:
Examiner registration number:

Baby AP (anteroposterior)

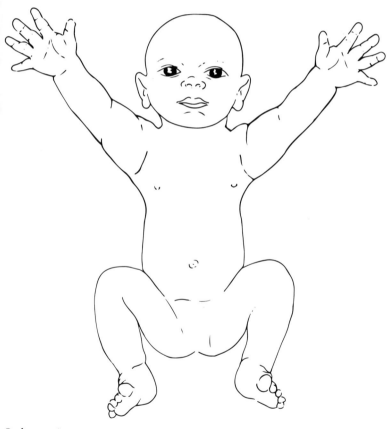

Body map 1

Patient Name:

Hospital Number:

NHS Number:

Date of Birth:

Date of Examination:

Examiner:

Examiner registration number:

Baby PA (posteroanterior)

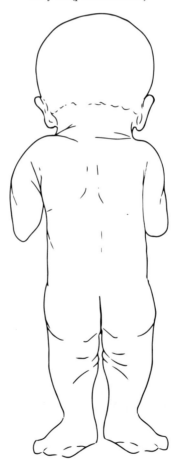

Body map 2

Patient Name:
Hospital Number:
NHS Number:
Date of Birth:
Date of Examination:
Examiner:
Examiner registration number:

Baby left lateral

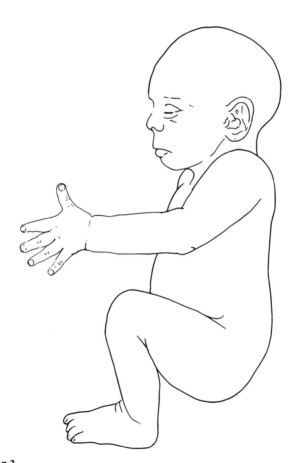

Body map 3

Patient Name:
Hospital Number:
NHS Number:
Date of Birth:
Date of Examination:
Examiner:
Examiner registration number:

Baby right lateral

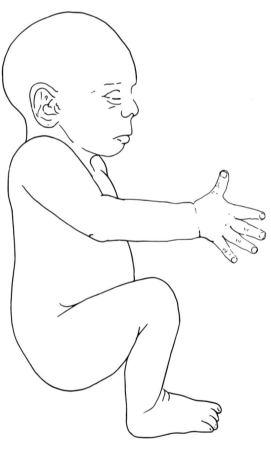

Body map 4
Copyright © 2015 Conrad von Stempel

Patient Name:

Hospital Number:

NHS Number:

Date of Birth:

Date of Examination:

Examiner:

Examiner registration number:

Toddler AP (anteroposterior)

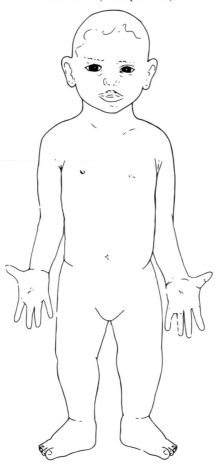

Body map 5

Patient Name:

Hospital Number:

NHS Number:

Date of Birth:

Date of Examination:

Examiner:

Examiner registration number:

Toddler PA (posteroanterior)

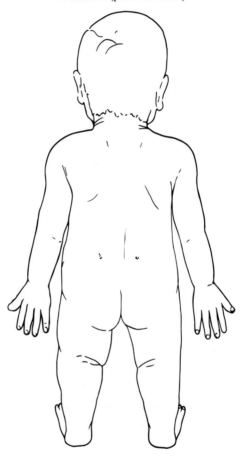

Body map 6

Patient Name:

Hospital Number:

NHS Number:

Date of Birth:

Date of Examination:

Examiner:

Examiner registration number:

Toddler left lateral

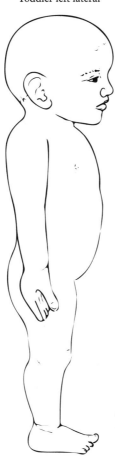

Body map 7

Patient Name:

Hospital Number:

NHS Number:

Date of Birth:

Date of Examination:

Examiner:

Examiner registration number:

Toddler right lateral

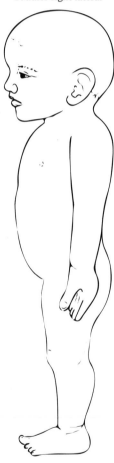

Body map 8
Copyright © 2015 Conrad von Stempel

Patient Name:

Hospital Number:

NHS Number:

Date of Birth:

Date of Examination:

Examiner:

Examiner registration number:

Young male child AP (anteroposterior)

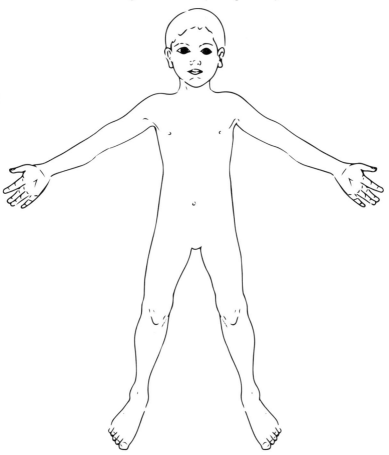

Body map 9

Patient Name:

Hospital Number:

NHS Number:

Date of Birth:

Date of Examination:

Examiner:

Examiner registration number:

Young male child PA (posteroanterior)

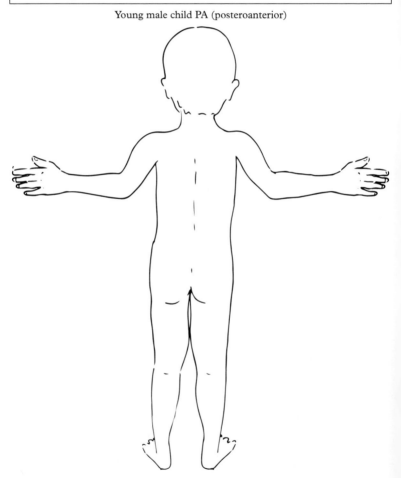

Body map 10

Patient Name:

Hospital Number:

NHS Number:

Date of Birth:

Date of Examination:

Examiner:

Examiner registration number:

Young male child left lateral

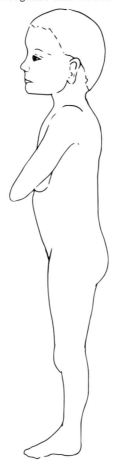

Body map 11

Patient Name:

Hospital Number:

NHS Number:

Date of Birth:

Date of Examination:

Examiner:

Examiner registration number:

Young male child right lateral

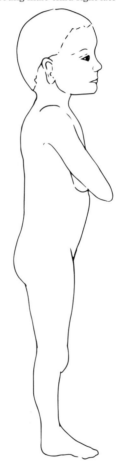

Body map 12

Patient Name:

Hospital Number:

NHS Number:

Date of Birth:

Date of Examination:

Examiner:

Examiner registration number:

Young female child AP (anteroposterior)

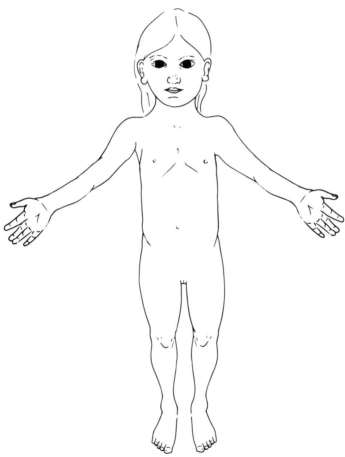

Body map 13

Patient Name:
Hospital Number:
NHS Number:
Date of Birth:
Date of Examination:
Examiner:
Examiner registration number:

Young female child PA (posteroanterior)

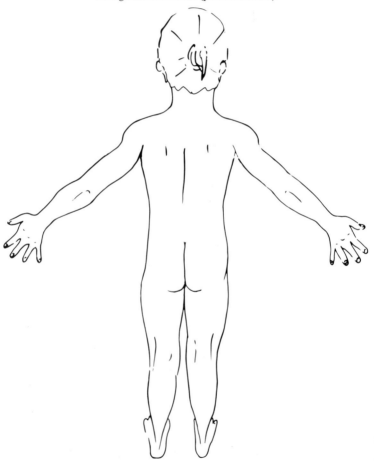

Body map 14

Patient Name:

Hospital Number:

NHS Number:

Date of Birth:

Date of Examination:

Examiner:

Examiner registration number:

Young female child left lateral

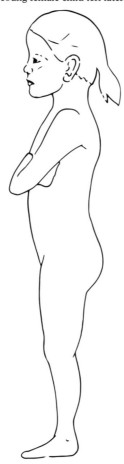

Body map 15

Patient Name:

Hospital Number:

NHS Number:

Date of Birth:

Date of Examination:

Examiner:

Examiner registration number:

Young female child right lateral

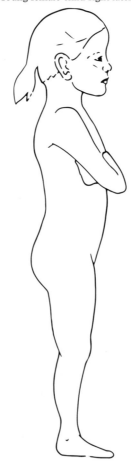

Body map 16

Copyright © 2015 Conrad von Stempel

Patient Name:

Hospital Number:

NHS Number:

Date of Birth:

Date of Examination:

Examiner:

Examiner registration number:

Male teenager AP (anteroposterior)

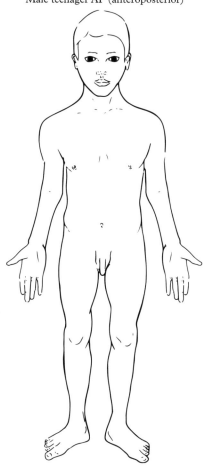

Body map 17

Patient Name:

Hospital Number:

NHS Number:

Date of Birth:

Date of Examination:

Examiner:

Examiner registration number:

Male teenager PA (posteroanterior)

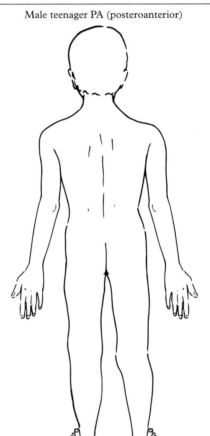

Body map 18

Patient Name:

Hospital Number:

NHS Number:

Date of Birth:

Date of Examination:

Examiner:

Examiner registration number:

Male teenager left lateral

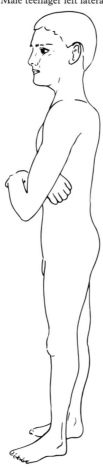

Body map 19

Patient Name:

Hospital Number:

NHS Number:

Date of Birth:

Date of Examination:

Examiner:

Examiner registration number:

Male teenager right lateral

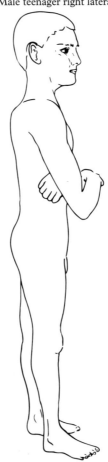

Body map 20

Patient Name:

Hospital Number:

NHS Number:

Date of Birth:

Date of Examination:

Examiner:

Examiner registration number:

Female teenager AP (anteroposterior)

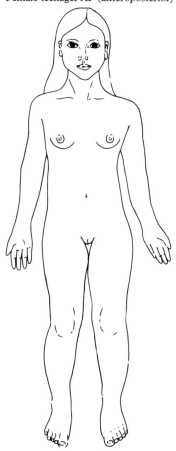

Body map 21

Copyright © 2015 Conrad von Stempel

Patient Name:

Hospital Number:

NHS Number:

Date of Birth:

Date of Examination:

Examiner:

Examiner registration number:

Female teenager PA (posteroanterior)

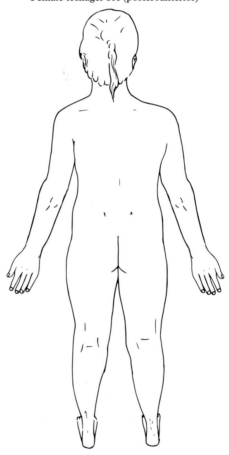

Body map 22
Copyright © 2015 Conrad von Stempel

Patient Name:

Hospital Number:

NHS Number:

Date of Birth:

Date of Examination:

Examiner:

Examiner registration number:

Female teenager left lateral

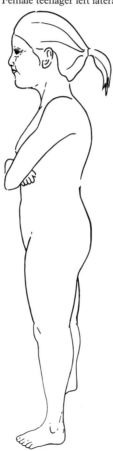

Body map 23
Copyright © 2015 Conrad von Stempel

Patient Name:

Hospital Number:

NHS Number:

Date of Birth:

Date of Examination:

Examiner:

Examiner registration number:

Female teenager right lateral

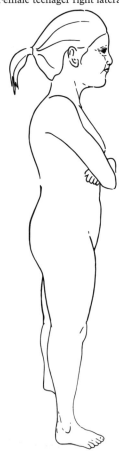

Body map 24

Patient Name:

Hospital Number:

NHS Number:

Date of Birth:

Date of Examination:

Examiner:

Examiner registration number:

Scalp (skyline view)

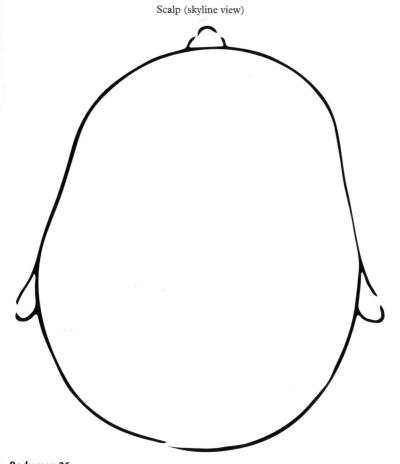

Body map 25
Copyright © 2015 Conrad von Stempel

Patient Name:

Hospital Number:

NHS Number:

Date of Birth:

Date of Examination:

Examiner:

Examiner registration number:

Eyes

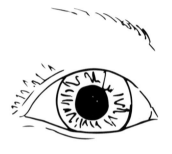 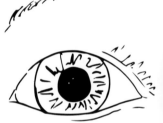

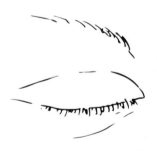 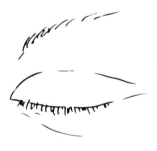

Body map 26
Copyright © 2015 Conrad von Stempel

Patient Name:

Hospital Number:

NHS Number:

Date of Birth:

Date of Examination:

Examiner:

Examiner registration number:

Frenuli

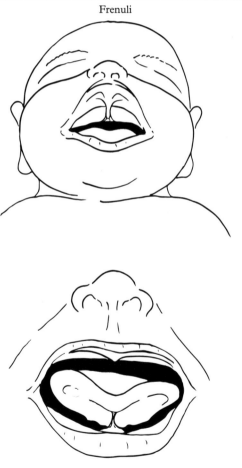

Body map 27
Copyright © 2015 Conrad von Stempel

Patient Name:

Hospital Number:

NHS Number:

Date of Birth:

Date of Examination:

Examiner:

Examiner registration number:

Left ear

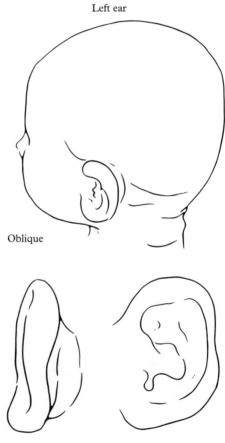

Oblique

Posterior auricular   Lateral

Body map 28
Copyright © 2015 Conrad von Stempel

Patient Name:

Hospital Number:

NHS Number:

Date of Birth:

Date of Examination:

Examiner:

Examiner registration number:

Right ear

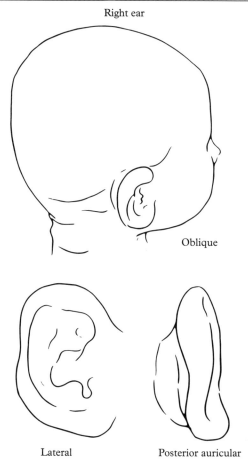

Oblique

Lateral

Posterior auricular

Body map 29

Patient Name:

Hospital Number:

NHS Number:

Date of Birth:

Date of Examination:

Examiner:

Examiner registration number:

Left hand and axilla

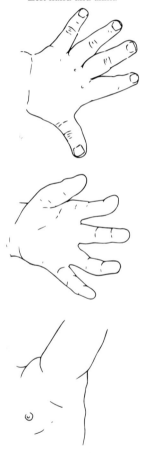

Body map 30
Copyright © 2015 Conrad von Stempel

Patient Name:

Hospital Number:

NHS Number:

Date of Birth:

Date of Examination:

Examiner:

Examiner registration number:

Right hand and axilla

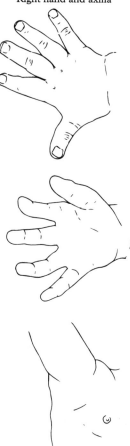

Body map 31

Patient Name:

Hospital Number:

NHS Number:

Date of Birth:

Date of Examination:

Examiner:

Examiner registration number:

Male and female genitalia

Female

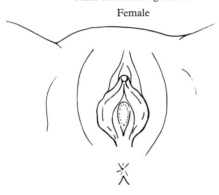

Male - lateral

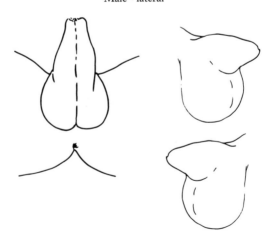

Body map 32
Copyright © 2015 Conrad von Stempel

Patient Name:

Hospital Number:

NHS Number:

Date of Birth:

Date of Examination:

Examiner:

Examiner registration number:

Feet dorsal surface

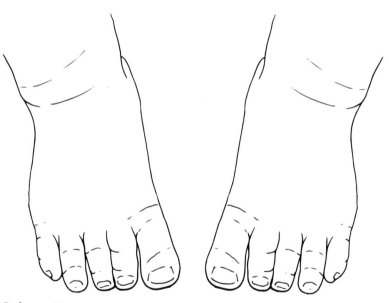

Body map 33
Copyright © 2015 Conrad von Stempel

Patient Name:

Hospital Number:

NHS Number:

Date of Birth:

Date of Examination:

Examiner:

Examiner registration number:

Feet plantar surface

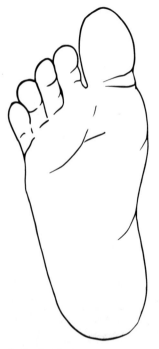
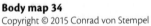
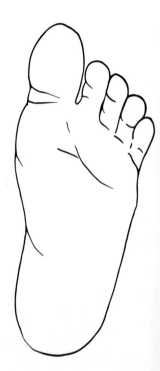

Body map 34
Copyright © 2015 Conrad von Stempel

Appendix 7

Discharge planning meeting proforma

Gayle Hann

Discharge Care Plan/Discharge Planning Meeting Summary

Name of Child:	
Child's DoB/EDD:	
Address:	
Hospital no:	
Hospital consultant:	
Whereabouts of child (if born, which hospital and ward is caring for the child):	
Is child subject to CP plan (Y/N):	
Is child subject to any legal orders (Y/N) (please state):	
Parents' details (please include both mother and father if known):	
Parental responsibility:	
Contact telephone numbers:	
Details of significant others:	
Specify any known risks:	
PROFESSIONALS INVOLVED:	
Details of social worker/team involvement (where appropriate):	
1. **Name, agency contact details:**	

2. Name, agency contact details:

3. Name, agency contact details:

Emergency duty team: (tel. . . ..)

GP details:

Health visitor:

School:

Reason for referral to social care:

Outcome of social work referral (to be completed by social worker):

Action to be taken at birth/discharge and by whom (social worker needs to consider):

◆ Is baby/child subject to CP plan?

◆ Can baby stay with its mother if not what is the plan?

◆ Is a discharge planning meeting needed? (A DPM must take place if the baby/child is subject to a CP plan)

◆ Is there a medical plan in place (if applicable)?

◆ Can the baby/child be discharged with the parent/s?

◆ Paediatrician to be informed: name of consultant/date/time.

Discharge address (include foster carer details and address/unit address):

Are parents aware of this plan (if NO, explain why):

Plan prepared by: (name, role, and contact number)

Date:

Plan agreed by: (name, role, and contact number—if meeting, attendees sign here)

Date:

Reproduced with the permission of North Middlesex University Hospital's Child Protection Team

Index

Note: Tables, figures, and boxes are indicated by an italic *t*, *f*, and *b* following the page number.